Health Care of the Aged: Needs, Policies, and Services

The *Journal of Gerontological Social Work* series:

- *Gerontological Social Work Practice in Long-Term Care*, edited by George S. Getzel and M. Joanna Mellor

- *A Healthy Old Age: A Sourcebook for Health Promotion with Older Adults (Revised Edition)*, by Stephanie Fall Creek and Molly Mettler

- *The Uses of Reminiscence: New Ways of Working with Older Adults*, edited by Marc Kaminsky

- *Gerontological Social Work in Home Health Care*, edited by Rose Dobrof

- *Gerontological Social Work Practice in the Community*, edited by George S. Getzel and M. Joanna Mellor

- *Social Work and Alzheimer's Disease: Practice Issues With Victims and Their Families*, edited by Rose Dobrof

- *Ethnicity and Gerontological Social Work*, edited by Rose Dobrof

- *Gerontological Social Work With Families: A Guide to Practice Issues and Service Delivery*, edited by Rose Dobrof

- *Gerontological Social Work: International Perspectives*, edited by Merl C. Hokenstad and Katherine A. Kendall

- *Twenty-Five Years of the Life Review: Theoretical and Practical Considerations*, edited by Robert Disch

- *Health Care of the Aged: Needs, Policies, and Services*, edited by Abraham Monk

Health Care of the Aged: Needs, Policies, and Services

Abraham Monk
Editor

The Haworth Press
New York • London

Health Care of the Aged: Needs, Policies, and Services has also been published as *Journal of Gerontological Social Work*, Volume 15, Numbers 3/4 1990.

The Haworth Press, Inc., 10 Alice Street, Binghamton, NY 13904-1580
EUROSPAN/Haworth, 3 Henrietta Street, London WC2E 8LU England

Library of Congress Cataloging-in-Publication Data

Health care of the aged : needs, policies, and services / Abraham Monk, editor.
    p. cm.
    "Has also been published as Journal of gerontological social work, volume 15, number 3/4, 1990" — T.p. verso.
    Includes bibliographical references.
    ISBN 1-56024-065-2 (alk. paper)
    1. Aged — Medical care — Government policy — United States. I. Monk, Abraham.
    [DNLM: 1. Health Insurance for Aged and Disabled, Title 18. 2. Health Policy — United States. 3. Health Services for the Aged — United States. W1 J0669NS v. 15 no. 3/4 / WT 30 H4342]
RA564.8.H4253   1990
362.1'9897'00973 — dc20
DNLM/DLC
for Library of Congress

90-4941
CIP

Health Care of the Aged: Needs, Policies, and Services

CONTENTS

ABOUT THE EDITOR

Abraham Monk, PhD, is Professor of Social Work and Gerontology at the Columbia University School of Social Work in New York City and Director of the Institute on Aging at Columbia University. He also served as Associate Director of the Long Term Care Gerontology Center of Columbia University's Faculty of Medicine. Prior to his affiliation with Columbia University, he was Professor of Social Work at the State University of New York in Buffalo and Director of its Multidisciplinary Center on Aging.

Dr. Monk is the author of over 100 publications in refereed scholarly and professional journals, as well as chapters in several books in the field of aging, social planning, and evaluative research. He is also the author of four books including *Resolving Grievances in the Nursing Home* (Columbia University Press). The revised, second edition of his *Handbook of Gerontological Services*, will be released in Spring 1990. Dr. Monk is the editor of a series of books titled the *Columbia Series of Social Gerontology and Aging*, launched in 1983 by Columbia University Press. He has conducted extensive research on intergenerational relations, housing and sheltered environments, long term care, pre-retirement preparation and post-retirement adjustment, and policy formation concerning families of the aged. He has recently conducted a study of home care services in six countries, with a grant from the USDHHS-Administration on Aging.

Dr. Monk is a Fellow of the American Gerontological Society and served as its Vice President. He received numerous awards including Fulbright Senior Scholarship and has served as consultant to many international, national, governmental, and voluntary service organizations in the field of aging. He received his undergraduate education at the National University of La Plata (Argentina) and his graduate degrees from Columbia and Brandeis Universities.

Health Care of the Aged: Needs, Policies, and Services

SYSTED 91 - SYSTEMS SCIENCE IN HEALTH-SOCIAL SERVICES FOR THE ELDERLY AND THE DISABLED

First Announcement
Fourth International Conference
Barcelona Palace of Congress
June, 10-14, 1991

The International Institute for Systems Science in Health Care announces SYSTED 91, an international scientific conference about problems connected with the health and social services for the elderly and the disabled.

The objective is to address the problems of planning, organization and management of health and social services for the elderly and the disabled. These problems are so complex, that very often no single discipline or profession can solve them satisfactorily, and a multidisciplinary approach is needed.

SYSTED is made up of systems scientists, professional providers and policy makers, interacting with a focus of advancing research and planning on behalf of the elderly and disabled.

The first SYSTED conference was held in Montreal in 1983, the second, in Perth (Australia) in 1987, the third in Bologna (Italy) in 1990.

Deadline for abstracts or sessions proposals: 31 December 1990.
Mail to:

World except North America:

Dr Josep Mª Via i Redons
Department de Salut Púlica
i Legislació Sanitària.
Unitat de Medicina Preventiva.
Divissiò Ciències de la Salut
Facultat de Medicina (Annex
Farmàcia)
Avgda, Diagonal, s/n
(Pedralbes)
08028 BARCELONA
PHONE: 343-339.11.11
(ext. 224)
FAX: 343-490.49.09

North America:

Dr. Charles Tilquin
Department d'Aministration de
la Santé.
Faculté de Medicine.
Université de Montréal
EROS/DASUM
C.P. 6128, Succ. A
Montréal, Québec
Canada H3C 3J7
PHONE: 1-(514)-343-5973
FAX: 1-(514)-343-2207

For more information: INTER-CONGRES
Gran Via de les Corts Catalanes, 646
08007 BARCELONA
PHONE: 93-3012577
FAX: 93-3016332

About the Contributors

JAMES J. CALLAHAN, JR., PhD, is Director of the Policy Center on Aging at the Florence Heller Graduate School for Advanced Studies in Social Welfare, Brandeis University, in Waltham, Massachusetts.

CAROLE COX, DSW, is Associate Professor at the National Catholic School of Social Services, The Catholic University of America, Washington, DC.

STEPHEN CRYSTAL, PhD, is Chair of the Division on Aging, Institute for Health, Health Care Policy and Aging Research, of Rutgers University, in New Brusnwick, New Jersey.

GERALD M. EGGERT, PhD, is Executive Director of the Monroe County Long Term Care Program, Inc. East Rochester, New York.

BRUCE FRIEDMAN, MPH, is Director of Research and Planning, Monroe County Long Term Care Program, Inc. East Rochester, New York.

MARYLOU GUIHAN, MA, is Project Manager at the Center for Health Services and Policy Research, Northwestern University, Evanston, Illinois.

SUSAN L. HUGHES, DSW, is Director of the Program in Gerontological Health, Center for Health Services and Policy Research and Associate Professor, The Medical School of Northwestern University, in Evanston, Illinois. Dr. Hughes is also Health Services Research Coordinator at the Lakeside Veterans Administration Medical Center in Chicago, Illinois.

LENARD W. KAYE, DSW, is Associate Professor at the Graduate School of Social Work and Social Research, Bryn Mawr College in Pennsylvania.

xiii

PATRICIA M. KIRWIN, PhD, is Lecturer at the Graduate School of Social Work and Social Research, Bryn Mawr College in Pennsylvania.

ABRAHAM MONK, PhD, is Professor of Social Work at the Columbia University School of Social Work, in New York City.

PHYLLIS MUTSCHLER, PhD, is Senior Research Associate at the Florence Heller Graduate School for Advanced Studies in Social Welfare, Brandeis University.

F. ELLEN NETTING, PhD, ACSW, is Associate Professor in the School of Social Work, Arizona State University, Tempe, Arizona.

CYNTHIA STUEN, DSW, is Director of The Lighthouse National Center for Vision and Aging in New York City.

JAMES G. ZIMMER, MD, is Associate Professor in the Department of Community and Preventive Medicine, School of Medicine and Dentistry, University of Rochester Medical Center, Rochester, New York.

Preface

Some time ago Abe Monk and I participated together in a workshop on the occasion of the celebration of the 90th Anniversary of the Columbia School of Social Work. The exact title of the workshop has escaped my memory, but it had to do with health care for the aged, and both Professor Monk and I were impressed by the number of CUSW alumni who chose our workshop, and also by the range and the depth of their interests in the subject.

There was no reason to believe that the interest of our participants that day was not shared by their colleagues in other cities, and so we concluded that a special volume devoted to policy and service issues in health care for the elderly would be in order. Professor Monk agreed to edit the collection. Herewith the fruits of that conversation, and of Professor Monk's labors and the labors of the extraordinary group of authors he was able to recruit to the task.

With pride I commend this collection to you: I believe Professor Monk chose the critical content areas, and chose also the best possible people to write about them. The first article, which Professor Monk authored, is required reading, I believe, for all of us who are concerned about "Health Care for the Aged," and also is an essential backdrop for the rest of this volume. Each of the papers merits a careful and reflective read, and Professor Monk, the authors, and I would welcome comments from our readers.

Rose Dobrof

Health Care for the Aged:
The Pursuit of Equity
and Comprehensiveness

Abraham Monk

SUMMARY. A quarter century after Medicare's enactment, the initial expectations of its gradual transformation into a comprehensive national health program did not materialize. The opposite is the case, as the federal government seeks to further curb its fiscal liability in health care. Demographic pressures exacerbate, however the demand for services. Planners responded to this demand with efficiency related strategies, but services remain inadequate and inequitable. The Catastrophic Coverage Amendments were repealed precisely because of their perceived built-in inequitable financing. A new policy agenda will emerge focused on home care alternatives to institutionalization, and long term care initiatives.

MEDICARE, THE DRGs AND THE MARKET ECONOMY

The aged are caught in the sweeping, almost cataclysmic changes currently occurring in the financing, organization and delivery of human and health care services.

It is a far cry from the optimistic climate of the early sixties when Medicare surfaced as the first federally sponsored health insurance program for the 65 plus population. Medicare signaled then the beginning of a new ideological posture in public responsibility. True, it was limited to a single age cohort but its advocates made no secret what their real intentions were: they expected Medicare to become the pilot or harbinger of no less than an all-encompassing national health insurance program. Wilbur Cohen, one of the main architects

---

An earlier version of this paper was presented at the Columbia University School of Social Work, Ninetieth Anniversary Celebration, October 14, 1988.

1

of the Medicare and Medicaid legislation, made no bones about his philosophical commitment to a comprehensive nationwide health insurance plan (1985). (He admitted, however, it had little chance of being adopted and that it would be more judicious to follow an incremental approach as was previously the case with Social Security.) He consequently suggested the creation of Medicare as early as 1950, as a fall back position after the defeat of Truman's more universal national health insurance proposal.

Given thus the incrementalistic nature of America's policy making processes, those advocates assumed that once a compartmentalized program like Medicare was set in place, resistances against a broader form of national health insurance would weaken. Medicare's extension to other age groups would then be only a matter of time.

A quarter of a century later it is more than obvious that the agenda in question did not materialize. In fact, the opposite may well be the case, as Medicare has turned into an embattled program, overwhelmed by a siege mentality due to the federal government's unmistakable decision to further curb its fiscal liability in the human services field. Services, most especially health care, are now treated like any other commodity in the open market.

The pendulum of governmental responsibility has, therefore, swung from one end to the other, but it is not devoid of a certain degree of ambiguity and contradiction. Altman and Rodwin observe that government regulations and competitive markets co-exist side by side in the health care field, with neither of these strategies for allocating medical services actually taking the lead (1988). Government would like to see a market economy flourish, but it persists in its determination to shape and oversee the operation of the market in question.

One recent manifestation of budgetary regulation—Medicare's prospective payment system—establishes a compensation rate for each of about 476 diagnosis related groups or DRGs. There is evidence that it produced short run improvements in hospital management, but its driving force has been cost containment rather than consumer choice, as would befit a market economy. Hospitals may be reaping greater revenues, but it remains to be proven whether costs will be brought under control. The savings realized by the DRGs may ultimately have to be applied to finance more outpatient and home care services, as well as to respond to the increased pressures for earlier admissions to nursing homes. Furthermore, accessibility has hardly improved under the new DRG provisions. A study by Carroll L. Estes of a random sample of about 800 community providers in five states revealed that almost half of hospital discharge planners reported experiencing difficulties in linking patients to community services (1988). Moreover, the community services networks have become "saturated" with more difficult, frail patients in need of more intensive and complex care. The allegation that Medicare patients are being discharged "sicker and quicker" remains, however, inconclusive. Mayer-Oakes et al. compared Medicare and non-Medicare patients, collecting data on treatment intensity and post hospital disposition. Hospital length of stay decreased substantially for both groups even among seriously ill patients who were admitted to the medical intensive care units, but they did not observe significant increases in-hospital or six-months mortality rates (1988).

From a budgeting standpoint, the percent of the GNP consumed by health care continues to inch up slowly but relentlessly, from 7.7 percent in 1972 to 11.2 percent in 1987 and, the DRGs notwithstanding, it may reach the 15 percent mark by the year 2,000. It was only 3.5 percent in 1929!

This increase in costs may be attributed to such factors as the utilization of a more complex technology, the employment of more sophisticated multidisciplinary teams of primary, secondary and tertiary providers, the practice of a more "defensive" form of medicine and the skyrocketing costs of malpractice insurance.

Inflation has also been historically more pronounced in the health and human services. It must be recalled that since hospitals were reimbursed for all reasonable costs they had no incentive to save. Finally, there is the sheer demographic expansion in the use and demand for services.

THE DEMOGRAPHIC BACKGROUND

The demographic factor enters here as the most decisive variable. It may be redundant to go over the obligatory recitation of facts and figures but it is an inevitable prerequisite for a practice and policy discussion to highlight the main trends. To begin with, it is already commonplace knowledge that life expectancy is steadily increasing: more people live longer and the proportion of older persons relative to the total population is also expanding; women outlive men and more older persons live alone.

The widowed older person, regardless of sex, tends to live alone rather than in a family setting. In 1950, only one in every seven lived alone; 30 years later, in 1980, the percentage doubled to nearly 30 percent, or one in three, approximately. As it may be surmised from the disparity in marital status of older men and women, there are also substantial differences in the living arrangements of the two groups. Out of the above mentioned group—the 30 percent who live alone, or a total of 8 million in 1982—most are women. Only 14 percent of the older men live alone, compared to 40 percent of the women. Of those 75 and older, half of the women and about 20 percent of the men live alone (U.S. Bureau of the Census, 1982, 1983), but very few of the aged live in multigenerational households. Caregivers of those who are frail and dependent must, therefore, shuttle between two home settings and manage both of them, a fact that adds to the sheer physical exertion and the strain of their supportive duties.

The most critical demographic issue is the higher survivorship in the 75 and older group. Family caregiving is more than a sporadic event. It has virtually turned into a continuous, indefinite and protracted correlate of women's life experience. The cause is primarily but not exclusively a demographic one. Between 1960 and 1970 the population 75 years of age and older grew at a pace three times as great as the 65-74 cohort. While less than 5 percent of the population was 75 or older in 1982, by the year 2030 and at the above mentioned rate, almost 10 percent of the total population is expected to be in that age group. Moreover, the population that is 85 years and older constitutes today about 1 percent of the total population—some 2.2 million. It will proportionately increase fourfold by 2030, thus taking a 4 percent share of the projected population. It is mindboggling to observe the skyrocketing increase in this latter group, from a total of 123,000 in 1900 to 2.2 million in 1980, and to a projected 16 million by 2050 (U.S. Bureau of the Census, 1981).

Because older age is associated with higher rates of illness and disability, the increasing numbers of very old people would be expected to lead to substantial increases in multiple chronic conditions and disability rates. The Health Interview Survey of 1981 confirmed that the mean number of bed-disability days per year was 11.5 for the 65-74 cohort (National Center for Health Statistics, 1981). For the 75 and older group the average climbed by 70 percent to 18 days. Hospital usage also increased with age. Discharge rates for persons over 85 years of age are 77 percent higher than for the 65-74 age group (National Center for Health Statistics, 1982:2).

THE EPIDEMIOLOGICAL BASE OF SOCIAL POLICY

James Fries advanced the "compression of morbidity" hypothesis, based on an examination of epidemiological trends in age and disability rates (1980). Fries contends that life expectancy will eventually plateau and cease in its relentless ascent, while chronic impairments will surface later and later in life. Rather than experiencing a slow, gradual decline that begins in early adulthood and stretches for three or four decades, people will — on the average — enjoy full or nearly full functional capacity until reaching advanced old age and then, they will almost suddenly experience a terminal drop and die.

Tracy did not find support, however, for Fries' hypothesis (1987). By comparing ADL scores — that is functional measures of activities of daily living performance — gathered in three national studies, the National Survey of the Aged (1962) and the National Health Interview Surveys of 1977 and 1984, she observed that there is a pronounced increase, not a decline — as anticipated by Fries — in disability rates. For instance, the percentage of 85 years of age and older who are dependent in mobility, who have difficulty in walking or transporting themselves rose from 19.2 percent in 1962 to 50 percent in 1984. Schneider and Brody similarly observed that disability rates increase in earlier cohorts, those in their sixties and seventies, not only those in their eighties (1983).

Whatever side we take concerning the "compression of morbidity" hypothesis, what really matters, from a policy and service delivery perspective, is the sheer numerical weight of surplus disability resulting from higher survivorship rates. Even if assuming that Fries is right, he would have proven that there is a relative postponement of disability in an individual's life cycle, but the aggregate effect of so many more older people living longer, into their eighties, would still be a steady demand for a complex and costly battery of service supports.

It is here where policy analysis can help to understand what it is that older people need, expect or demand from the helping professions. Historically, research on both community based and institutional services started out with inquiries on the patterns, frequencies and outcomes of service utilization behaviors among the aged.

This research consisted of the usual count of visits to physician's outpatient clinics, lengths of stay in hospitals, rehospitalization rates, frequencies and ranking of diagnostic categories, and determinants of the transition from hospital and community, to lengthier or permanent institutionalization. It began with an epidemiological model and it moved into the incorporation of social and psychological interpretative models. It eventually fanned out into a series of parallel investigative tracks.

First, as government became more cost conscious, the political economy of health care came to the fore with the analysis of the adequacy and complementarity of public and private programs designed to provide such care.

Second, the political economy perspective also opened the door to ethical, philosophical and legal questions about equity and limits in the provision of care. Researchers asked about the extent of society's responsibility in the provision of care for the aged, and what arrangements ought to be made for the benefit of a larger number of beneficiaries. They also raised these ultimate and inescapable questions: services for what purpose? Are they meant to prolong life or to also enrich it? Do the services succeed in fostering a better adjustment to the aging process?

Third, health promotion and resocialization programs raised optimistic hopes that older persons could successfully neutralize decompensating processes and even regain functional abilities through systematic behavioral changes. The ensuing evaluative research did not render, however, simple answers about the legitimacy or validity of those contentions.

Fourth, evaluative research was associated with at least two additional areas:

a. The impact of the service system on the aged as consumers; the consideration of their needs and preferences and the extent to which they participate in decisions affecting the course of care; their ultimate satisfaction with the care they receive and their compliance with programs designed to enhance their functional independence.

b. The planning and structural considerations about the access to service programs and their coordination in more effective and efficient packages. Let us keep in mind that we have only recently witnessed the experimentation with demonstration and pilot projects, such as HMOs, S/HMOs, single entry points, case management and so on. They are still being tested and reviewed.

HEALTH SERVICES UTILIZATION: NEEDS AND PATTERNS

Older persons double or nearly double the rates of chronic conditions afflicting the succeeding cohort of middle agers, those 45 to 64 years of age. In the case of arthritis, it is 443 per thousand people 65 and over, as compared to 253 people 45 to 64. A similar pattern is seen with heart illness (274 versus 128 per thousand); visual impairments (118 versus 58); diabetes (80 versus 58), and hypertension (385 versus 214 per thousand) (National Center for Health Statistics, National Ambulatory Medical Care Survey, 1981). It is not surprising that older persons have higher rates of physician contacts but they are far from doubling that of younger age groups. In 1983 the average number of these contacts was 7.6 per year per person, as compared to 5.0 visits for persons of other age groups. Older persons have greater reliance on the direct relationship with their physicians, at the doctors office, but rate below the total population in their utilization of hospital outpatient departments. Physician visits have remained on the average fairly constant over the last 20 years, despite the near universal enrollment in part B of Medicare. They barely increased from 6.7 visits in 1964 to the already mentioned rate of 7.6 in 1983 (U.S. National Center for Health Statistics, 1983).

The elderly also use inpatient hospital services with greater frequency than any of their succeeding age cohorts. Granick and Short found that persons aged 65-79 spent on the average almost 11 days in short term hospitals, a 30 percent increase over the 8.4 days for those 40-64 years of age (1985). Utilizing data from the Hospital Cost and Utilization project of the National Center for Health Services Research and Health Care Technology Assessment, Granick and Short further report that although the older group has a higher average number of diagnoses (3.1 versus 2.5), fewer surgical procedures are performed on this group (41.5 versus 52.2 percent). The differences widened when comparing discharge rates: three times as many elderly as the middle agers 40 to 64 years of age are discharged from the hospital to another health facility, rather than to their homes in the community (6.3 percent versus 1.9 percent). This anticipates the inexorable role that long term care services begin to play among the old.

It is surprising to note, however, that the elderly have lower rates of admission to both inpatient and outpatient mental health services than virtually any other age group. Once again, it would be unwarranted to conclude that they experience lower rates of mental impairment. What seems to be at play, in the case of outpatient services, is that older persons tend to use their primary care physicians rather than psychiatrists, social workers or other professionals for their mental health needs. This is confirmed in a recent study by Carol E. Blixen (1987). Based upon private practice findings from the National Medical Care Survey (NAMCS) as well as on mental health visits to hospital clinics and emergency rooms in New York City during a three month period in 1984, Blixen observed that almost half of all visits to a physician, resulting in a mental disorder diagnosis were to non-psychiatrists.

Older persons appear in fact to be the lowest ranking consumers of private practice mental health services, barely 6 percent of all hospital ambulatory care visits made by their age group, as compared to 25 percent of all ambulatory care visits made by the 25 to 44 years of age group. A different picture emerges when observing hospital utilization rates. The 65 and older population made more intensive use of specialized psychiatric clinics than they did of general medical clinics. Medicare was more likely to be the payer when those psychiatric clinics were utilized. However, when the primary payer was other than Medicare, the greater number of mental health visits was made to general, non-specialty clinics.

This happened despite the greater flexibility and freedom of choice of mental health provider offered by the non-Medicare payers. It is not easy to interpret these intriguing practices. Blixen identifies two concurrent although not complementary patterns. The higher use of specialized mental health clinics may simply be the outcome of prevailing clinical referral practices. In other words, once the tranquilizers and antidepressants prescribed by primary care physicians are rendered ineffectual they have no other recourse but resorting to more specialized settings.

The elderly are also creatures of habit and when afforded the opportunity they would return for all their needs, including the mental health ones, to the general hospital's outpatient clinics and emergency rooms. They form over the years close attachments to their neighborhood hospitals and view them as their overall providers, not different from their local supermarkets. They prefer this "one step" medicine, even when their insurance allows them to seek out the services of more sophisticated and better equipped facilities.

DETERMINANTS OF SERVICE UTILIZATION

What conditions determine the use of health care services? The mere fact that persons suffer a debilitating illness, or realize that they are progressively deteriorating cannot guarantee that they will resort to available health services. Researchers have inventoried myriads of variables that correlate and affect both utilization rates and utilization patterns. Andersen and associates developed probably the most widely used conceptual model that aims to systematize and integrate all potential factors (1973). It classifies the variables in three major groups:

1. *predisposing*, that is, social structural elements such as ethnicity, religious beliefs, cultural norms and family attitudes;
2. *enabling*, comprehends personal circumstances such as in-

come, transportation and geographical location that may facilitate or hinder the use of a given service, and

3. *need* factors, which include subjective feelings and perceptions of one's own disability.

Petchers et al. studied access to health care in a black urban elderly population (1988) and concluded that enabling variables do make a difference. Affordability was a major barrier to medical care for this group of poor minority aged. Despite their high rates of enrollment in Medicare, — virtually the same for all the aged — they experienced psychological distress because of the difficulty in meeting the increasing costs of care: virtually no one had transportation problems and could reach health facilities fairly easily. Most respondents had a particular health facility or hospital as the regular place of care. However, the lack of a regular physician conspired against the continuity of care and turned it into a major source of frustration and dissatisfaction. The authors hypothesize that the mechanisms that link the individual to the health care system are as important as the service itself and they surmise that the concept of availability may have to be divided into two components: *first*, the availability of the service itself, and *second*, the availability of continuous physician care, and where rapport between professional provider and consumer can gradually develop into a personalized relationship.

An important and intriguing study about this physician-elderly patient relationship and communication was completed by E. Brody (1985). Health professionals she surveyed were of the opinion that older persons interpret physical and mental ailments as normal concomitants of the aging process, and resign themselves to conditions that could actually be reversed. The aged become victims of these self-fulfilling prophecies and regard it pointless to consult health specialists once their chronic conditions have been diagnosed.

Older persons tend to confide their physical symptoms to relatives and other professionals but conceal, or at least withhold information, about emerging mental deficits and emotional concerns. They also believe that practitioners are not interested in their elderly patients, and that they are imbued of what is known as "therapeutic nihilism," that is, a sense of futility as far as aiming to bring about cure, recovery or restoration of function. Moreover, the aged respondents are by and large convinced that the health professionals rarely tell them the truth about their conditions and future prospects. Paradoxically, older persons are satisfied with the professional care they receive but they condition it to an honest exchange, and a good explanation of their condition given by the practitioner. It would appear that aged patients value good rapport as much as the possibility of cure.

One of the most singular findings in Brody's study relates to the stereotype of older persons as cantankerous and habitual complainers, given to fill their time with anxious phone calls to their physicians to report all sorts of real or imaginary aches and pains. The opposite appears to be the case. The aged underreport and even conceal their symptoms, including those that are potentially serious. They would rather endure them with fortitude. It does not mean that the aged do not seek relief but this is frequently requested from their informal network, rather than from professionals. They resort to nonprescription drugs or share prescription drugs that may have worked for a friend, spouse or relative. They also tend to ignore treatments prescribed by their physicians claiming they induce adverse effects, or because they disagreed with the regime altogether.

Older persons wish for the most part, to receive complete explanations of the causes and nature of their ailments, the reasons for whatever treatment is prescribed and its chances for success. They want the opportunity to remain in some control, to ask questions, express reservations and inquire about alternatives.

Good rapport and communication between providers and consumers of service will not, however, always result in better treatment compliance. People do not always act in their health's best interest. Some knowingly persist in self-destructive behaviors. Furthermore, no healthy life style and systematic prevention can avoid the risk of certain conditions. Senile dementia, just to cite one, will affect one out of every 20 older Americans, or about 4 million people by the turn of the century. There is a danger that this realization may lead to discouragement and the rejection of preventive intervention and programs. It is the "what is the use" excuse for not participating, but there is also the danger that too much emphasis on preventive care may deflect attention from the shortcomings of the present health system and assume, as some have interpreted Fries theory, that in the long run there will be a need for less, not more services. It is here where questions concerning the adequacy of the present service system come to the fore.

ADEQUACY AND EQUITABLE ACCESS

Health and social services for the aged have evolved in the U.S. without the benefit of previously thought-out blueprints or master plans. They resulted instead from expedient policy reactions to public clamor and circumstantial political agendas. Over the years, and since the passage of the Social Security Act in 1935, more than 250 programs of national scope have been mandated by federal policy. We would like to understand them as constituting a *de facto* continuum, ranging from health and social services for the "well," to those for the severely decompensated aged, in need of round-the-clock long term care services. They were not conceived, however, as a coherent system or continuum. Services are fragmented and reveal gaps: some needed services are hardly available while others do not meet the volume of need.

From a policy and planning standpoint one may question how well the services in reference meet the manifest needs of the aged and also how accessible they are to them.

Let us examine this latter issue of accessibility: to begin with, older persons need more than one service at any given time, yet different service providers must attend to separate eligibility rules. The multiplicity of these rules alone acts as a barrier that discourages service utilization. Furthermore, for over thirty years the United States followed an income rather than a service strategy toward the aged. There is no service tradition altogether as far as the aged are concerned. It was only in 1964 that the Older Americans Act (OAA), was passed to foster the coordination of services and the development of gap-filling new services. As a result of the OAA, the integration of services was conducted through more than 600 Area Agencies on Aging. Some are coterminous with a single city or county, others like Nevada covered an entire state. They instituted single entry points, up-to-date information and referral services and the planning of community and concrete social services. They usually do not provide any major direct service, save for nutrition. Their handicap is that they are mandated to coordinate services over which they have little or no statutory authority, especially over health services, and they can hardly use the leverage of budgetary allocations because, except for nutrition funds, they have little funds to allocate. Their impact on the health care system is rather minimal. The health system falls, for the most part, outside the OAA's domain, which means that there are virtually two contiguous, parallel but poorly related service systems.

A different approach to service coordination and accessibility that encompasses more effectively the health care system evolved from case management experiences. These have been initially tested in a number of "channeling" projects fostered by the Health Care Finance Administration over the past decade. Case managers assess the problems and needs of the elderly patients; they determine the range of services needed, consult with a team of assorted providers—both within and outside the hospital; they negotiate and advocate with other health and social service providers to ensure that services will be delivered as scheduled; they monitor and reassess the condition of the patient and eventually prescribe and oversee a new cycle of services.

Case management is the inevitable corollary of an age of service specialization and of a service system which does not facilitate easy access. Case management is a service that helps precisely in reaching other services. It does not, however, create by itself those other services when they do not exist. It seeks to ensure accessibility amidst conditions of service selectivity. This is both its strength and its weakness. There is no conclusive evidence of its effectiveness, but, on the other hand, there are no alternative models of procurement or linkage to services, that have proven to be effective either.

There is an ethical dimension to service accessibility that has not escaped the attention of policy analysts. It centers around the concepts of "equity" and "fairness." They imply among other, the means and ways to ensure the reasonable and adequate provision of services at a cost that does not constitute an excessive or impossible burden. The debate around what constitutes fair charges for a given service, what are the limits in catastrophic situations beyond which individuals or their families should not be required to slide into total impoverishment, and who should ultimately foot the bill is still raging.

It was originally assumed that Medicare would automatically resolve the "equitable" access problem, at least for older Americans. After all it extended health coverage to millions of elderly who formerly had no insurance protection. For a short while the policy worked, as evidenced by the marked reduction in death rates among the elderly. Medicare assured in principle, the right to health care, but it did not extend it to all types of care and wavered about the extent to which older persons would share in the costs.

Medicare was a good beginning but it failed the moral test of equitable access. Many policy analysts take, in retrospect, an "I told you so" posture. Laura Katz Olson, for instance, contends that Medicare was superimposed on an "unresponsive," profit-motivated and privately-controlled hospital market (1982). Its emphasis on acute illness and hospital-based care was a consequence, according to Rich and Baum, of Congress' eagerness to mollify the American Medical Association (1984). Hospital care was forced upon the elderly population without consideration to other probably more needed and less expensive community and home based services.

Medicare gave preference to technological and hospital based services but neglected prevention, rehabilitation and home care services. Olson added that it fostered the "exploitation of illness" for profit, thus enhancing the power and economic rewards for the provider; it also promoted greater institutionalization, which in turn produces the systematic pauperization of the aged; and finally it focused attention on medical services without consideration of the social and environmental causes of ill-health and dependency.

It may be added that Medicare fostered an overreliance on specialists but failed to reward the attention to older patient's overall concerns. It depersonalized the treatment relationship because it was more concerned with symptoms than with the patients' feelings.

Above all, Medicare failed to cover the full or most of the costs of illness. The aged had to participate with a vast array of deductibles, exclusions and cost sharing provisions that increase year after year, usually at rates higher than the increase in the cost of living index. The result was that the elderly were forced to pay an increasingly greater share of their health bills, and Medicare paid, in turn, only 44 percent of the health costs of the aged. Even if including Medicaid, which accounts for another 15 percent, the aged are still responsible for approximately 40 percent of their total health bill. To protect themselves from the eventualities of catastrophic illness, about one half of the aged have purchased costly private supplementary insurance, but many of these policies are virtually useless given their severe restrictions of benefits. At best they cover only 5 percent of the health bill.

Despite the large budgetary outlays earmarked for Medicare and Medicaid, there has not been a redistribution of health services that takes into account the risks and needs of the mainstream of older persons, those who are not rich enough to face any eventuality, but are not yet totally destitute as to qualify for Medicaid.

THE PURSUIT OF EQUITY

There are three policy trends dominating the latter end of the 80s. They are the dominant initial agenda for the 1990s.

The first has already been manifested in the recently enacted and almost immediately repealed Medicare Catastrophic Coverage Act of 1988. It was the largest single expansion of Medicare in its 24 years of existence. The provisions of the bill were meant to be phased in over three years and would have included unlimited hospital coverage beyond an annual deductible of about $600.

Substantial gaps remained, however. It did not cover much needed and costly dental services and hearing devices, physician charges that exceed the limit set by Medicare, and extended indefinite stays in nursing homes, actually the greatest source of catastrophic expense for older Americans.

The 1988 amendments adopted, on the surface, an unmistakably redistributive approach toward the financing of health care for the aged. It aimed to ease the costs of medical care for low income elderly and, conversely, increase them for the more affluent elderly. Basically, the aged would have to bear the entire bill on their own. The reality is, however, that there are not too many rich older persons. The higher costs would have descended on persons of modest resources. It would have taken an income of approximately

$27,500 in 1989 to become liable for the maximum additional individual tax of $800. Critics of the new catastrophic provisions have therefore denounced it as an escalating and confiscatory tax, ironically adopted at a time when tax rates for the higher income brackets of the American population were being considerably reduced. Moreover the new law promised coverage that many elderly felt they were already receiving at a lesser cost through Medigap insurance policies. Also, as pointed out by H. T. Steve Morrisey, on behalf of the National Association of Retired Federal Employees (1989), the provision of extended hospital care is of little or no consequence because hospitals rarely keep a patient for more than sixty days. If a patient needs such prolonged treatment, in all likelihood it is of a maintenance nature and the hospital will then require his or her transfer to a nursing home or a similar long term care facility. This was precisely one of the main shortcomings of the Catastrophic bill: it steered away from long term care, even if between 20 and 40 percent of all elderly will eventually need institutional services.

Second, simultaneously with the preceding Medicare Catastrophic Act of 1988, the House of Representatives considered HR 3436, the Medicare Long Term Home Care Catastrophic Protection Act, better known as the "Pepper bill." This proposed legislation was better attuned to the long term, chronic care needs of millions of incapacitated and disabled persons of all ages, not only the elderly. It centered around the provision of an assortment of long term home health services and the training of primary support networks, so that relatives and other caregivers could assume a more effective role in attending to the needs of older patients. It also fostered a series of demonstrations that would test the feasibility of adult day care services for both the physically incapacitated, and the seriously mentally ill. Conscious of the imperative of fiscal restraint and aiming not to add to federal deficit, the Pepper bill proposed a self-financed package of services. These would be paid by eliminating the $45,000 ceiling on earned income which is currently subject to social security taxes. Such change would affect only about five percent of the nation's wage earners, those in the higher income brackets. It would thus turn around an unfair regressive tax and make it precisely more progressive.

The Pepper bill was defeated mainly because of bad timing, as its vote almost coincided with the passing of the Catastrophic Coverage Act. There was an awareness in Congress even before its repeal, that the Catastrophic Coverage Act fell short of the mark and needed to be supplemented with legislation which is more responsive to the growing demands for long term care. This is evidenced by the fact that Congress created a bipartisan commission to recommend alternative directions for comprehensive and long term care, as a follow up of the Pepper bill's debate.

The third and final major area of policy consideration concerns the role that long term care insurance may play to finance nursing home care. The costs of these services will continue to escalate and will pass the 100 billion mark by the turn of the century. A study by Alice Rivlin and Joshua Wiener under the auspices of the Brookings Institution indicates that private insurance initiatives will not suffice to finance long term care (1988). Most such policies offer fixed indemnity benefits which will easily erode even under mild inflationary conditions. Moreover, they tend to require prior hospitalization as a condition of eligibility, when it is known that only 39 percent of current admissions to nursing homes originate in hospitals. A tax financed public insurance program will have to be implemented for the long haul, that is, for those who are institutionalized for more than the three years of benefits offered by most private programs. Public insurance may, therefore, act as a residual program picking up from the point of termination of the private sector's products. The public program will be covered, as suggested by Rivlin and Wiener, by Medicare, that is, by a social insurance mechanism, and not by Medicaid, which is essentially a welfare program.

Policy analysts forecast the inevitable explosion in the demand for long term home care services. Area Agencies on Aging surveyed in 1985 after the implementation of DRG provisions indicated a 196 percent increase in skilled health care in the home and a 69 percent increase in housekeeping or homemaking. Length of service and number of services per client increased for most agencies where DRGs had been in effect. The cost containment provisions inherent to the DRGs shift a major portion of the burden of health care away from acute care hospitals to the community based care systems. These, however, are not properly in place nor have adequate provisions for the funding been made so far. The policy agenda points in the direction of long term care, both community and institution based. It will be expensive but inevitable and everybody will have to pay for it.

The argument that the younger generations are getting restless and tired of paying more social security taxes to take care of the growing number of older persons is contradicted by every public opinion poll conducted in the last decade. A national survey recently conducted by Louis Harris found that 82 percent of the American people could not afford paying for long term care, whether at home or in a nursing home, but over 80 percent of the same respondents supported the idea of a federal long term care insurance program for the aged and the chronically ill (1988). Also, 70 percent of the same sample favored a specific tax to finance the federal long term care program.

Independently of these trends in federal legislation, states have already begun containing the growth and even reducing the number of both acute care hospitals and institutional facilities. New York State has been encouraging, in turn, the expansion of home care and has called for increasing by 100 percent the number of certified home health agencies.

In sum, the Medicare Catastrophic Coverage Act of 1988 contained some laudable provisions but did not address the main health concerns of the aged. It imposed an onerous and inequitable new tax but offered too little in return. It remained "specialist" oriented, like the original Medicare, and largely side-stepped the multiple needs which afflict the chronically ill, that is, those who require long term, continuous care. It is not surprising therefore that the aged did not rally to the support of the bill, despite appeals from the leadership of the American Association of Retired Persons. Their membership simply did not follow them.

Medicare was an auspicious beginning in health insurance but it has not yet produced an equitable and comprehensive health care system for the aged. Whether future policy developments will be circumscribed to the aged and selected target groups, or will instead be subsumed under a wider and far reaching national health insurance program remains, for the moment, a matter of speculation.

This is the challenge that will dominate the health policy agenda of the 1990s.

REFERENCES

Altman, S.H. and Rodwin, M.A., 1988. "Half way competitive markets and ineffective regulation: the American health care system." *Journal of Health Politics, Policy and Law* (Summer), 13, (2), 323-339.

Andersen, R. and Newman, J., 1973. "Societal and individual determinants of medical care utilization in the U.S." *Milbank Memorial Fund Quarterly*, 51, 95-124.

Blixen, C., 1987. "The ambulatory care setting as the mental health service provider to older adults." Doctor of Philosophy Dissertation, Heller School, Brandeis University, Waltham, Mass.

Brody, E.M., 1985. "Mental and physical health practices of older people." Springer Publishing Company, New York, NY.

Cohen, Wilbur J., 1985. "Reflections on the enactment of Medicare and Medicaid," *Health Care Financing Review*, Annual Supplement, 3-11.

Frics, J.F., 1980. "Aging, natural death, and the compression of morbidity." *New England Journal of Medicine*, 1980, vol. 303, 130-135.

Granick, D.W. and Short, T., 1985. "Utilization of hospital inpatient services by elderly Americans." DHHS Publication (Public Health Service 85-3351). National Center for Health Services Research.

Harris, Jr., L., 1988. Testimony (March 29), in "The need for long term care: a survey of public opinion." Hearings before the Subcommittee on Health and Long Term Care, House Select Committee on Aging, Washington, DC.

Katz-Olson, L., 1982, "The political economy of aging." Columbia University Press, New York, NY.

Mayer-Oakes, S., Oye, R., Leake, B., Brook, R.H., 1988. "The early effect of Medicare's prospective payment system on the use of Medicare intensive care services in three community hospitals." *Journal of the American Medical Association*, December 2, 260 (21), 3146-3149.

Morrisey, H.T.S., 1989, Letter to the editor in "Catastrophic health act punishes the elderly," *The New York Times*, July 24, 1989, A16.

National Center for Health Statistics, "1981 Health Interview Survey." (unpublished).

National Center for Health Statistics. "1981 National Ambulatory Medical Care Survey." Reported in the U.S. Senate Special Committee on Aging; *Aging America*, 1984 edition.

National Center of Health Statistics, 1982, "The need for long-term care: a chartbook of the Federal council on the Aging and the 1981 National Hospital Discharge Survey," in Special Senate Committee on Aging, Developments in Aging 1.

National Center for Health Statistics, "Health Interview Survey, 1983." Reported in U.S. Senate Special Committee on Aging; *Aging America*, 1985-86 edition.

Petchers, M.K. and Milligan, S.E., 1988. "Access to health care in a black urban elderly population." *The Gerontologist*, April, 28 (2), 213-217.

Rich, B.M. And Baum, M., 1984. "The aging: a guide to public policy." University of Pittsburgh Press, Pittsburgh, PA.

Rivlin, A.M. and Wiener, J.A., 1988. "Caring for the disabled elderly." The Brookings Institution, Washington, D.C.

Schneider, E.L. And Brody, J.A., 1983. "Aging, natural death and the compression of morbidity: another view." *New England Journal of Medicine*, Vol. 309, 854-856.

Tracy, K.B., 1988. "Trends in personal care dependency in the older population: 1962 to 1984," Doctor of Public Health Dissertation, School of Public Health, Columbia University. New York.

U.S. Bureau of the Census, 1981. "Projections of the population of the United States: 1982-2050." Current Population Reports 25 (Middle Series Projections; #922).

U.S. Bureau of the Census, 1982. Current Population Survey (March 1982).

U.S. Bureau of the Census, 1982. "Marital status and living arrangements." Current Population Survey (March 1981) Series P-20 (372).

U.S. Bureau of the Census, 1983. Current Population Survey (March 1983). (unpublished).

Health Economics, Old-Age Politics, and the Catastrophic Medicare Debate

Stephen Crystal

SUMMARY. For several decades old age benefits saw maintenance of previous gains and periodic improvement in scope. Political accommodations "spread the wealth" to prosperous and poor aged, to health providers and other stakeholders, finessing legislative roadblocks and financing conflicts, but demographic and health economic trends suggest an end to this era. Medicare Catastrophic repeal epitomizes health policy stalemate, presaging a more conflictual era in the 1990s. Divergent economic interests among subgroups of elderly and inflationary economics of fee-for-service medicine are subtexts to the debate suggesting that future benefits expansion will be elusive and that lesser structural reforms in the health care system can be implemented.

In the mid-1960s, in a step perceived by many of its advocates as a way-station to a universal national health insurance system, Congress enacted the Medicare program. The financial commitment entailed in this step far outstripped expectations, with the resulting cost overruns a major obstacle to the hoped-for extension of publicly funded care to other age groups. Nevertheless, the basic structure of Medicare benefits remained stable over the years. The long-standing consensus over the program's financing, however, was sharply interrupted in the controversy surrounding the passage, and, late in 1989, the repeal of the package of benefit expansions encompassed in the "catastrophic coverage" amendments. These benefits were to have been financed, in part, by the introduction of an income tax surcharge, with some surcharge being paid by approximately 40 percent of the elderly (those with higher income tax liabilities), and the maximum surcharge being paid by 5 to 10 percent of the best-off elderly.

It has become increasingly apparent that we have entered a period of difficult choices in paying for health care for the growing elderly population, with conflict over who should pay for these benefits becoming increasingly overt and divisive. Medicare costs have been growing at a rate far exceeding the rate of inflation—sixteen times, in fact, since the late 1960s. Growth substantially exceeding inflation has been true in the hospital sector even though the introduction of the diagnostic-related group system has slowed the growth in Part A from what it would have been without prospective reimbursement (Russell, 1989). It has also been true in the area of physician services; the consumer price index for such services increased by 359 percent in the 20 years following 1967, as compared with 240 percent for the all-items CPI (National Center for Health Statistics, 1989). While hospital charges were the fastest-increasing medical prices during the 1970s and early 1980s, price increases for physician services have outstripped them since 1985 (National Center for Health Statistics, 1989).

The crisis in Medicare reflects a more basic watershed in American health care politics. Improvements in coverage in the past have typically been achieved by a process of compromise which accommodated all interest groups and overcame provider objections by sufficiently sweetening the deal for them. This process, however, now seems unviable in the face of the seemingly uncontrollable economics of the U.S. health care system.

This system is in many respects a unique phenomenon. Its delivery and financing structures differ from those in most industrialized countries, where some sort of national health system is the norm. The system also poses issues quite different from those faced in our own past, because the nature of health care has changed so dramatically and so quickly. It has been said that it was not until about 1940 that the average patient had much chance of benefiting from an encounter with the average physician. Penicillin, the first major antibiotic, was a World War II innovation. Even as recently as the mid-1960s, the scope of what medical care could do was dramatically less than today. In 1965, health spending, at $205 per capita, was less than 6 percent of gross national product (National Center for Health Statistics, 1989). As one evidence both of the cost of the system and of our failure to provide full protection even to the best-insured age group in our society, the elderly are now paying more of their income for health care than they did before the enactment of Medicare in the mid-1960s—an average of $1,055 per capita in 1984 excluding long-term care costs (Owens, Oberg and Polich, 1988), and dramatically higher for the chronically ill needing long-term care.

The catastrophic insurance debate was somewhat catastrophic for the aging community, since it divided many constituencies who previously have made common cause toward improving services to the elderly. On one side were many people of good will who saw it as a great accomplishment that an additional level of protection was provided to those who incur extremely lengthy hospital stays or very high physician or pharmaceutical bills, even if the legislation did not address the more important problem of long-term care. Many of these people felt it was quite appropriate, given recent trends in the economic status of the elderly, for the higher-income elderly to contribute to the cost on an income-related basis, which might well result in an individual paying more surtax than the benefit was worth to him or her. On the other side have been those who doubted the value of what was being provided (particularly for those who already had private insurance supplements), who questioned the redistributional aspect of the financing, or who challenged the precedent that Medicare enhancements be financed from within the elderly population itself. While the original debate was complicated and technical, once the bill was passed and individuals could assess what it meant to them personally, many of the more articulate and influential of the elderly found they were going to be paying substantial sums for benefits to which they attached little value or which duplicated coverage they already had.

This catastrophic insurance debate is a harbinger of challenging times in aging policy, times which will force us to confront difficult choices in a harsher fashion than previously characteristic of modern American old-age policy, in which continuing incremental improvement has been the norm ever since the 1930s. The dissension reflects difficult underlying issues. One such subtext is the widespread perception that our medical care system is not producing value for money. Physician costs are currently a source of particular concern for policymakers and the public generally; they increased from $8.5 billion in 1965 to $92 billion in 1986, with 29 percent of the cost (as compared with less than 10 percent of hospital cost) being borne directly by the patient (Health Care Financing Administration, 1987). As with hospitals before prospective reimbursement, physicians have done well under the Medicare system which organized medicine originally opposed vehemently. Income after expenses for all U.S. office-based physicians averaged $119,500 in 1986 and $132,000 in 1987 (American Medical Association, 1988). The planned implementation of a Relative Value Scale for physician reimbursement may redress the imbalance between reimbursement for cognitive and for procedural medical services, and could create the potential for longer-term savings, but at least in its initial implementation it is intended to be cost-neutral, reflecting the continuing pattern of Congressional compromise with health care providers which has been believed to be necessary to enact each reform in Medicare.

What individual health care consumers see at their own personal level, health care analysts see at the system level. Because of its unique political history, the American health care system in recent decades has tended to socialize the financing of care while privatizing the delivery system. For years, open-ended reimbursement systems, oriented to fee-for-service payment, increased demand for care while insulating providers from market forces which would otherwise constrain the prices they could command. The results were massive health care inflation, with the consumer price index for all medical services increasing by 400 percent during the 1967-1987 period, a rate of increase 166 percent that of the all-items index (National Center for Health Statistics, 1989). Increasingly, the structural divergence of the American health care system from that of other developed countries — its diverse, open-ended, and fee-for-service orientation — has been joined by a cost divergence as increasing shares of U.S. gross national product are committed to health care. The share of US gross national product devoted to health care has risen from less than 6 percent in 1965 to over 11 percent today (Letsch, Levit, and Waldo, 1988). In Western Europe and Canada, where there are national health systems and national coverage, health care costs range from 6 to 9 percent of GNP. For example, Great Britain in 1986 spent 6 percent and West Germany 8 percent (Relman, 1989).

The sense that the health care marketplace is out of control, and dominated by powerful provider forces who have arranged matters so that they are immune both from the laws of supply and demand that constrain prices in the rest of the economy and from centrally imposed budgets, is one reason why it is difficult to achieve consensus on who should pay. Another subtext is the divergence of economic interests and health care concerns and interests within the elderly population. One reason that many of the better off elderly opposed improving the publicly funded system is that so many of them have privately purchased coverage for those costs, and many others have supplemental coverage at no cost to themselves through former employers.

Analysis of the relationship of economic status and health status among the elderly, and the distribution of health insurance coverage, sheds light as to this divergence of interests within the elderly population.[1] This analysis, utilizing data from the 1984 panel of the Census Bureau's Survey of Income and Program Participation (for a description of SIPP, see Herriot and Kazprzyk, 1986), shows that the high-income elderly are more likely than those with low income to have coverage which supplements the basic Medicare benefits. In addition, the coverage is more comprehensive—for example, it is more likely to cover physician costs, not just those for hospitals, not covered by Medicare.

In this analysis, elderly respondents were ranked by overall economic well-being into quintiles. The measure of economic well-being used in the analysis, documented in detail by Crystal and Shea (1989), adjusted each respondent's household income for household size, for underreporting of some types of unearned income characteristic of this and other Census data sets, and for the annuitized value of assets. This process allowed us to assign elderly respondents to categories according to a broader measure of eco-

1. The contribution of Dennis Shea in the analysis of the SIPP data is gratefully acknowledged.

nomic well-being than that afforded by the use of personal or household income alone.

Among respondents in the top quintile, 72 percent had supplemental coverage in their own name, versus only 40 percent of those in the lowest quintile. The disparity was even sharper when coverage of non-Medicare eligible physician charges was examined: the best-off were more than twice as likely to have such coverage in their own name (58 versus 28 percent). Even more dramatic was the fact that the best-off were more than 6 times as likely to be covered by another's insurance, since even when household size is adjusted for, the poor elderly are likely to be widowed or single while the best-off are more likely to be married. The poorest were three times as likely as the well-off elderly to be reliant on Medicare alone, without supplements, to pay for their health care, even accounting for those with access to Medicaid. The comfortable asset position of those likely to pay the maximum surtax, those in the top quintile, also suggests their lack of dependence on Medicare alone, with average adjusted net worth of more than $300,000.

Equally striking was the fact that the elderly most troubled by health problems and those who would have been subject to the catastrophic-care surcharge were quite different populations. Those in the top quintile averaged only 60 percent as many days of hospital care and 80 percent as many physician visits in the previous year as those in the lowest. They were less than half as likely to have vision problems and less than half as likely to have difficulty lifting ten pounds. They were only one-quarter as likely to report being in poor health status.

These findings suggest the divergence in economic and health-care interests between subgroups of the elderly which constituted one of the important subtexts of the catastrophic insurance controversy. These divergent interests now tend to divide the poor from the prosperous elderly, and those with chronic illness from those, particularly the "young-old," in relatively good health. The commonality of concerns once assumed can no longer be counted on.

In relatively homogeneous countries like those in Scandinavia and Western Europe, it has been easier in social welfare to build a consensus behind redistributional approaches to social insurance. In this country, that has been a more difficult political message to sell, and one current symptom of this aspect of our political culture is the reluctance of higher income elderly to cross-subsidize the poorer elderly's catastrophic Medicare costs. The data described above suggest that the bulk of the best-off elderly (those who would have been subject to the maximum surtax) have to a large extent been able to "opt out" of full dependence on the publicly funded Medicare system; have considerable ability to pay privately for any non-insured costs; and are in generally good health status, with less short-term likelihood of heavy health care bills. These elderly are also, by virtue of their income, education, and social standing, the most likely to wield political influence, and did so effectively in the catastrophic insurance debate.

In the light of these sources of contention in the politics of Medicare, what problems do future efforts to extend Medicare's scope face? While many advocates of repeal of the catastrophic insurance provisions argued that the absence of long-term care coverage was a principal reason for their opposition, the same divergence of interests which helped bring about the repeal will exist with respect to long-term care coverage. Further, if the present burgeoning of private long-term care insurance continues—a development encouraged by many, including federal spokespersons, as an "off-budget" means to fund care and control medicaid costs—we are likely to see a similar pattern of "opting out" of dependence on public programs by the best-off elderly. The widespread "in-principle" support expressed for improvement of public long-term care programs could well be thinner than expected, once the price tag is more apparent and once private alternatives are better-established. Since new revenues will probably be needed to fund new long-term care benefits—and since the elderly most in need of such services are least likely to be able to afford new financial burdens—equity considerations will once again suggest income-related cost-sharing. Such proposals, however, may face opposition from higher-income elderly similar to that encountered by catastrophic insurance. Funding through general tax revenues, given the resistance to new taxes and projections for continuing budget deficits, would spread the burden across generations. However, since the elderly have reached and perhaps passed economic parity with the non-elderly, on average, and are doing substantially better on average than children

(Hurd, 1989; Crystal and Shea, 1989), the resistance to such funding could well be substantial. Further, the problems of diverging interests and of "opting out" affect willingness to pay for such benefits not just by the high-income elderly but by the high-income middle-aged.

For the less well-off elderly, who live close to the economic margin, not only long-term care costs but also uninsured costs of acute illness continue to create the possibility of economic disaster. Costs of supplemental coverage are widely expected to increase by substantial percentages in the wake of repeal, further exacerbating the problem of affordability for supplemental coverage by this group. The subtexts of conflict between provider and beneficiary concerns on the one hand, and of conflict among beneficiary interests on the other, challenge our sense of community and require that we look much more sharply than we have had to do in the past at issues of burdensharing, of competition between differing interests, and of equity. The increasing divergence in health care costs between the United States and industrialized nations with national health systems suggests the acute need in this country to address basic questions of structure and organization in the health care system, of provider economic power in that system and of cost, as a prerequisite both to being able to think fairly about what the limits are and also as a prerequisite to being able to sell further benefit improvements to the taxpaying public. Data on the sharp economic inequality among subgroups of the elderly suggest the need to refocus our attention on the special problems of the elderly in greatest need, recognizing that meeting these needs requires acceptance of burdensharing by other constituencies, including the better-off aged.

There is widespread support in principle for improvement of coverage under Medicare, and extension of publicly funded care to other constituencies with special medical needs. The deleterious effects of lack of consistent access to prenatal and child health services have been well documented, generating substantial support for Medicaid expansions to include more of this population. New health care needs—for example, those of the growing HIV-infected population—are apparent. But the inflationary tendencies that appear to be built into our unique combination of extensive public funding and little public control of health care organization and delivery are becoming, even more clearly than before, the major obstacle to access improvements.

In this context, the catastrophic insurance fiasco can be seen as the paradigm of an era of "zero-sum health politics." Despite medical cost inflation, initiatives to address access problems—such as the extension of Medicare to kidney dialysis patients and the long-term disabled—have been possible periodically. But in the post-Reagan era of limited federal revenues and chronic budget deficits, general revenues did not appear to be a politically feasible route for the addition of catastrophic coverage, while the apparently ingenious surtax on upper-income elderly proved even less politically salable. The cost of additional benefits—which would go principally to chronically ill elderly who tend to be relatively poor—became a hot potato which the low-income elderly could not afford, the high-income elderly would not accept, and the Gramm-Rudmanized general revenue pool could not support.

The catastrophic Medicare reform experience has been interpreted in several ways. Some—occasionally using pejorative terms like "greedy geezers"—attributed its failure to an unreasonable reluctance by the high-income elderly to share their good fortune with the less-advantaged of their peers. Others argue that the fault was in departing from the tradition of funding Medicare through general taxation. Examination of Census income data suggests some of the reasons for political resistance to both of these financing routes. Many of the non-elderly lack enthusiasm for additional tax burdens to support medical care for a single age group whose average income no longer lags that of the non-elderly (Crystal, 1986; Hurd, 1989), given the unmet needs of other age groups. The relatively good health status and comfortable asset position of the high-income elderly, as well as their good private insurance coverage, suggests why they did not tend to value the new benefits highly. It is, then, not entirely surprising that this latest effort to enhance Medicare benefits hit the wall.

To some extent, of course, all social insurance programs involve "risk-spreading" and implicitly assume the subsidy of some classes of participants by others. However, it appears likely that the sources of dissensus over Medicare financing discussed above have been particularly insuperable because of the apparently uncontrollable nature of the increase in medical prices and the sense on the part of many consumers that the system is run, in many respects, by providers for the benefit of providers. These concerns become more apparent when an effort is made, as with the catastrophic insurance bill, to attribute particular taxes on particular beneficiaries to a particular set of incremental benefits.

In the political calculus, the crisis for consumers of uncovered and unaffordable health care costs can be seen as the thesis, and the "hot potato" syndrome in financing the heavy price tag for benefit improvements as the antithesis. What, then, is the synthesis? It is reasonable to suggest that a fundamental reconsideration of financing and reimbursement mechanisms under Medicare, and perhaps of the entire "supply-side" of traditional fee-for-service health care delivery, could emerge, as the only apparently feasible way to expand access without unmanageable cost. Extension of such structural reform to Medicare would parallel developments in employer-financed health care, where managed health care plans are rapidly displacing "traditional" indemnity systems. If—like Eastern Europe's economies—the political economy of U.S. health care has indeed reached a point of stalemate, and all roads now lead to system reform, then "relative-value" physician reimbursement could be only the beginning of rethinking accommodations enshrined in Medicare's structure for more than two decades.

REFERENCES

American Medical Association. *Socioeconomic Characteristics of Medical Practice*. Chicago: American Medical Association, 1988.

Crystal, S. "Measuring Income and Inequality Among the Elderly." *The Gerontologist* 26(1):56-59, 1986.

Crystal, S., Shea D. *The Economic Resources of the Elderly: A Comprehensive Income Approach*. Survey of Income and Program Participation Working Paper No. 89-14. Washington, D.C.: Bureau of the Census, 1989.

Health Care Financing Administration (Office of the Actuary). National Health Expenditures, 1986-2000. *Health Care Financing Review* 8(4), 1987.

Herriot R.A., Kasprzyk, D. *Some Aspects of the Survey of Income and Program Participation*. Survey of Income and Program Participation Working Paper No. 86-01. Washington, D.C.: Bureau of the Census.

Hurd, M. "Economic Status of the Elderly," *Science* 244:659-664, 1989.

Letsch, S., Levit, K., and Waldo, D. "National Health Expenditures, 1987." *Health Care Financing Review* 10(2):109-122, 1988.

National Center for Health Statistics. *Health, United States, 1988*. DHSS Pub. No. 89-1232. Washington: Government Printing Office, 1989.

Owens, S., Oberg, C.N., Polich, C. "Medicare Reform: The Emergence of Long-Term Care Proposals," Issue Paper No. 6, in Long-Term Care Expansion Program: Issue Papers, Volume 2, Excelsior, MN: Interstudy, 1988.

Relman, Arnold. "Confronting the Crisis in Health Care." *Technology Review*, July:31-40, 1989.

Russell, Louise. *Medicare's New Hospital Payment System: Is It Working?* Washington: Brookings, 1989.

Hospital-Based Long-Term Care Services for the Frail Elderly

F. Ellen Netting

SUMMARY. This paper examines acute care hospital diversification into long-term care services for the frail elderly. The discussion focuses on five multifaceted roles played by health care social workers as hospitals develop long-term care initiatives. The need for an advocacy stance in both macro and micro aspects of care is stressed. Ethical dilemmas that arise in hospital-based systems are presented.

INTRODUCTION

In 1918, World War I and epidemics of infectious diseases disrupted family life and employment for many. That same year, as medical social workers faced these challenges in the health care arena, they banded together to form a professional association through which practice wisdom and skills could be shared. Their response to urgent community needs and their desire for a professional approach to practice undergirded health care as a social work speciality. This speciality has continued to grow over the years (Kerson, 1979, p. 342).

Between 1960 and 1985 the number of social workers employed in health care settings in the United States doubled. Numbers are estimated at 45,000 (Berkman et al., 1985, p. 43). Today, over half of all health care social workers practice in acute care hospitals (Carlton, 1988). The social work education literature is filled with discussion regarding the integration of course content on social work practice in health care (Bennett & Grob, 1983; Bergstrom, 1979; Berkman, Kemler, Marcus, & Silverman, 1985; Borland & Strauss, 1982; Bracht, 1983; Lane, 1982; Wolkenstein & Laufenburg, 1981). Approximately half of all CSWE accredited schools of social work offer some form of health care concentration or specialization (Borland & Strauss, 1982 p. 225).

Working with frail older clients enmeshes the health care social worker in both acute and long-term care arenas. Programs in hospital in-patient and outpatient units, nursing facilities and home care environments require the practitioner to synthesize multiple perspectives as disciplines interact. The goal is to make sense of what is often a fragmented, complex delivery system so that older clients do not fall through gaps and become depersonalized. Even referring to this interactive dance as a system may be misleading because what occurs is often far from systematic. It is often the social worker who must attempt to make sense of the assortment of health care actors and plethora of services that older clients and their families encounter.

This paper examines the roles that health care social workers play in hospital-based long-term care programs designed for the frail elderly. Hospital diversification into geriatric long-term care begins our discussion. Ethical dilemmas that arise in carrying out social work roles will be examined, along with implications for social work practice in hospital-based settings.

HOSPITAL DIVERSIFICATION
INTO LONG-TERM CARE

In 1967, the National Commission on Community Health Services identified a growing need for long-term care and encouraged the building of "extended care facilities under hospital auspices as a national priority" (Prybil, 1980, p. 80). Potential benefits of hospital diversification into long-term care included economies gained in transferring patients from costly acute care to less expensive long-term care units, continuity of care for patients needing post-acute services, and the convenient on-site availability of specialized health care programs already offered by community hospitals and accessible to long-term care components (Prybil, 1980).

In recent years, hospitals have played a dominant role in health care provision for the elderly. Since the advent of Medicare, on average older adults have spent three times the number of days in hospitals as have adults in general. Approximately, 70 percent of Medicare dollars are used to cover hospital services (Eisdorfer & Maddox, 1988, p. 1).

> The largest group of hospital users, and the only group of high users that is going to grow for the balance of this century, is the elderly. Persons 65 and over already account for roughly 40% of all inpatient days in general hospitals . . . Thus the elderly are central to hospitals because they are the customers who consume the greatest single share . . . America's community hospitals are thus de facto geriatric institutions and will become more so, whether they know it or not. (Vladeck, 1988, pp. 38-39)

Acute care hospitals function within a rapidly changing health care environment. Recent trends have led hospitals to increasingly provide geriatric in-patient, post-acute and long-term care services. These trends include the growth of the older population in the United States; increased periods of disability due to technological advances to prolong life and the accompanying demand for longer periods of care; and changes in the structure of health care financing and organization (Capitman et al., 1988).

The latter trend was accentuated in October 1983 when the Health Care Financing Administration, some states, and some third-party payers began using diagnosis-related groups (DRGs) on which to base hospital reimbursement for inpatient care. This financing approach is based on the assumption that patients having similar medical conditions will need the same resources and require similar care. "Therefore, although there is a variation in resource consumption among patients within a DRG, this variation is expected to balance out across the range of all patients" (Graves, 1987, p. 1).

One strategy used by hospitals to adapt to this changing environment has been to develop new programs targeted to older persons and other users of long-term care. A 1985 American Hospital Association study found that 24 percent of the hospitals surveyed owned skilled nursing facilities, 12 percent owned intermediate care facilities, 33 percent offered home health services, 14 percent offered homemaker programs, and 2 percent provided specialty geriatric inpatient services (Read & O'Brien, 1986).

Southerland (1988) reports that Witt Associates, Inc. conducted a national survey of acute care hospitals and hospital systems with 300 or more beds to identify current and future long-term care plans. Forty-two percent of respondents indicated that they currently owned, leased or managed nursing homes. Asked about level of satisfaction with these new ventures, 26 percent reported that their nursing beds have exceeded expectations, whereas 60 percent felt their expectations were met but that improvements were still needed. Fifteen percent of respondents indicated that their hospitals were involved in the ownership, leasing, or management of one or more retirement communities. These ventures, however, were viewed with some uncertainty because of the potential risks involved. Eighteen percent of respondents had no plans to enter the retirement housing field in the future.

In some rural communities, which tend to have high proportions of older persons, hospital diversification into long-term care services has been used as a strategy to counteract low census rates in acute care beds. Bowlyow (1989), in her study of rural hospitals and long-term care service provision, found that smaller rural hospitals tended to have long-term care units. However, "the presence of LTC had no relationship to the percentage of elderly people in the community, suggesting that community need may not be an important characteristic" (p. 84). It is also important to distinquish between long-term care skilled nursing units and swing-bed programs which are Medicare reimbursed in rural hospitals of 100 beds or less (Williams, Netting, Hood-Szivek, 1988).

Although studies indicate increases in hospital diversification, not all hospitals have embraced long-term care services. Rocheleau (1983) explains why. First, a preoccupation with high technology and its accompanying status may cause community-based programs to take a 'backseat' to high-tech initiatives. Second, hospitals and existing community-based agencies have not always coordinated their efforts, thus creating a potential communication gap and a disincentive to work with other long-term care organizations in the community. In fact, there may be resentment toward the entry of hospitals into long-term care.

If hospitals, currently a major referral source for nursing homes, begin to provide long-term care services on a large scale, it will seriously threaten the success of the long-term care provider. In addition, hotel chains and housing developers can be formidable competitors in areas like senior housing and retirement centers. (Aiello, 1988, p. 25)

Third, older persons do not always embrace the idea of going to a hospital for services traditionally offered in less potentially threatening settings. In fact, hospitals are often perceived as institutions of last resort.

In those hospitals that do diversify into long-term care services, health care social workers are challenged to learn a new vocabulary. Older consumers are described as the "senior market" and "senior membership" programs are developed to entice consumers to one program over another. "Senior product lines" are discussed as hospital administrators and managers determine exactly what services will be developed and how they will be packaged. As diversification progresses, "vertical integration" occurs in which a continuum of needed acute and long-term care services are linked together to provide continuity of care. "Hospitals seeking vertical integration attempt to control, through ownership or management, all production and distribution processes directly related to their core activities" (Capitman et al., 1988, p. 21). Terms such as "managed care," "care management," and "case management" are used to describe oversight functions provided to facilitate the consumer through the system. Competition with other acute and long-term care systems will occur as each organization seeks to obtain its "market share."

SOCIAL WORK ROLES IN HOSPITAL-BASED LONG-TERM CARE

Given hospital diversification, and its accompanying jargon, what are the emerging services offered by hospital-based long-term care programs and what roles do social workers play within these initiatives? Five multifaceted, often overlapping roles are identified in Figure 1: (1) geriatric clinician, (2) transition manager, (3) post acute care provider, (4) chronic care specialist, and (5) geriatric educator. Selected hospital initiatives in geriatric long-term care are also listed in Figure 1.

Geriatric Clinician

The key social work role within the acute care hospital has remained essentially the same since medical social work was introduced into a Boston hospital in the early 1900s. The goals of hospital-based social work practice are twofold. First, the social worker assists the patient and his/her family in coping with the trauma and stress that precipitated the hospital visit. Second, the social worker must quickly, yet sensitively, facilitate decision-making and adaptation so that the patient achieves some mastery over what is happening (Bendor, 1987). This process usually begins at admission and continues throughout the patient's hospital stay.

Peterson (1987) provides a profile of hospital patients today.

Figure 1.

SOCIAL WORK ROLE	HOSPITAL-BASED INITIATIVES
Geriatric Clinician	o Geriatric Speciality Units o Geriatric Consultation Teams o Geriatric Outpatient Programs and Clinics
Transition Manager	o Discharge Planning o Short-Term Case Management
Post Acute Care Provider	o Skilled Nursing Facilities o Swing Beds o Step-down Units o Home Health Care o Hospice
Chronic Care Specialist	o Intermediate Care o Personal/Assisted Care o Adult Day Health Care o Home Aide/Homemaker o Long-Term Case Management
Geriatric Educator	o Geriatric Education o Support Groups o Senior Membership Programs o Respite Care

Given the number of out-patient procedures performed and the increasing pressures to discharge, Peterson tells us that

> inpatients found in the hospital today may be the people who were admitted at the last possible moment . . . They are sicker than the inpatients of the past, yet they have a shorter length of stay . . . [They] are older or at higher risk of complications . . . They are not the patients the hospital is attempting to attract. (pp. 4-5)

Therefore, the hospital-based social worker encounters patients who may have multiple needs, are particularly vulnerable, and are old.

The proportion of older persons within the hospital setting requires the social worker to have knowledge of aging and offers the opportunity to specialize in geriatrics. Hospital-based inpatient initiatives include specialized inpatient units, geriatric consultation teams, and geriatric outpatient programs and clinics. Geriatric speciality units are based on the British model of "progressive geriatric care." In the British system, older patients are immediately admitted to an acute-care geriatric assessment or evaluation unit where they receive a multidimensional, comprehensive assessment. Care plans are individually designed, based on data collected by an interdisciplinary team. Over the last ten years, the number of geriatric speciality units has been increasing in the United States as research studies document their effectiveness (Rubenstein, 1987).

The social worker who performs the geriatric clinician role serves multiple functions. These include: gatekeeper, advocate, interdisciplinary team member, psycho-social assessor, and facilitator in mastering illness and maintaining dignity.

Transition Manager

The transition manager is engaged in such services as discharge planning, and short-term case management. These roles have become more and more important as patients are readied for discharge as quickly as possible. The social work transition manager is in a unique position to provide oversight between the acute care episode and the patient's return to the community.

A recent longitudinal case study of a Minnesota hospital revealed that families of older patients are increasingly performing managerial roles post-discharge. With the implementation of DRGs, "it appears that families are more actively involved in managing post-hospital care and combining family-care with formally provided services" (Fischer & Eustis, 1988, p. 388). Social workers are trained in family dynamics and understand the concept of person-in-environment. Working closely with family support systems is a logical linchpin for the social work transition manager. It is important to recognize, however, that frail elderly patients do not always have family available, particularly family members who can provide care on an on-going basis. The social worker, therefore, is often an innovator—mobilizing informal support systems within the community to address client needs.

> Social work sees discharge planning as a complex service that requires rapid but accurate assessment of a multitude of social and emotional factors, an assessment of the adequacy of resources within the community, and an intervention designed to benefit the patient and his[/her] recovery. (Lawrance, 1988, p. 120)

In dealing with frail older persons, discharge planning becomes complicated when several services are needed to coordinate an adequate post-discharge plan, when family is either not available or nonexistent, when patients may disagree with medical advice, or when needed resources do not exist within the community. The literature provides numerous discussions of discharge planning and the social work focus in this transitional role (Blumenfield, 1988; Lawrance, 1988; Raush & Schreiber, 1985; Ritvo, 1988; Wolock et al., 1987) as well as the implications of discharge planning for client decision-making and self-determination (Abramson, 1988; Coulton et al., 1988; Dubler, 1988).

Often social workers have assumed that performing transitional roles such as discharge planning are too concrete and nonspecialized, thus having low status. Ballis (1985) points out that nurses have been quick to assume these roles and that health care systems depend upon this pivotal role in an environment that is predicated on efficient discharge. In addition, transition management "makes sense philosophically. The social work profession has always advocated for those that society often prefers to ignore: the sick, the poor, the elderly, the mentally disturbed, the developmentally disabled, and minority groups" (Ballis, 1985, p. 212).

Post Acute Care Provider

Health care social workers perform post acute care roles as well. These professionals work in hospital-based skilled nursing facilities, swing beds, step-down units, home health care, and hospice programs.

A study comparing hospital-based with community-based home health services revealed differences in client characteristics. Hospital-based clients were older and more functionally limited, thus requiring more intense services and a greater share of therapeutic activities. It was found that hospital-based patients tended to have been admitted to home health following an acute care episode more often than those persons receiving community-based home health services (Balinsky & Rehman, 1984). This study emphasizes the importance of understanding case mix in that hospital-based home health services may have frailer, more vulnerable clientele than their community-based counterparts.

Chronic Care Specialist

Hospitals began branching out into service areas that were the traditional domain of community-based networks. These services include intermediate care, personal/assisted care, adult day health care, home aide services, and long-term case management. The gerontological social worker hired by hospital-based long-term care programs may serve as a community liaison, supervisor of volunteers, and program coordinator.

Hospital-based long-term case management requires distinctly different activities from those performed by discharge planners, although these services are often confused and misunderstood. Whereas discharge planning ends as the patient exits the hospital, unless limited followup is scheduled, hospital-based case management is a long-term, post-hospital, intensive oversight process.

Simmons and White (1988) identify six case management functions: case finding, assessment, care planning, coordinating, followup, and reassessment. Various models of hospital-based case management primarily utilize social workers and nurses in a team approach.

Geriatric Educator/Advocate

Geriatric education and information approaches to hospital-based long-term care include lectures, support groups, senior membership programs and other related educational activities (Capitman et al., 1988). These hospital-based initiatives provide outreach into the community, opening hospital doors to professionals, paraprofessionals, and volunteers from diverse sectors.

Just offering these type services does not always assure success for the hospital system. One study of hospital-based respite care (Gonyea, Seltzer, Gerstein, & Young, 1988) found that simply making service available to caregivers of elderly residents would not assure service utilization. Respite care was to be viewed as an integral part of a treatment plan, rather than as an add-on service. The social worker's training in understanding systemic connections is particularly valuable in these type programs if they are to succeed as integrated parts of a continuum of care.

IMPLICATIONS

Hospital diversification into long-term care offers challenges and opportunities for the health care social worker. Not only are traditional inpatient roles available for social workers interested in working with the elderly, but hospital-based initiatives into post-acute and long-term care arenas require the performance of roles previously viewed as the domain of the "aging network" and its community-based providers.

A common thread throughout the five roles discussed is an overriding need for social workers to be advocates. The social worker, regardless of hospital-based setting, must constantly maintain a client advocacy stance. Otherwise, clients become lost in large hospital-based systems. This advocacy stance is manifested at both the macro and micro levels.

At the macro level, probably the most important thing the health care social worker can do in hospital-based programs is to assist in reframing how the system is perceived. Vladeck (1987) contends that the "dominant metaphors for continuum of care are misleading and potentially destructive" (p. 3). We view the continuum as a ladder, as concentric circles, and as a matrix.

The ladder metaphor places the intensive care unit of the acute hospital at the top because it requires the most comprehensive and skilled professional oversight. On the ground rung are in-home services. To illustrate how prominent this hierarchical continuum is, Vladeck reminds us of terms such as hospital "step-down" unit, vertical integration, higher and lower levels of care, and subacute care. This type of thinking drives the entire Medicare system in which a higher order of importance is given to certain services rather than others. The ladder concept derives from a medical model (Vladeck, 1987).

A second metaphor is a set of concentric circles. This model places the community hospital within the center circle, surrounded by circles of less intense levels of care. Vladeck (1987) explains that this metaphor

> continues to focus on moving clients among levels of acuity or intensity as if they were a kind of raw material flowing through an elaborate set of pipelines—indeed, *patient flows* is an invariably recurring phrase in discussions of this model. (p. 6)

A third metaphor is the three dimensional matrix. Vladeck explains:

> The axes are payment source, service mix, and site. Taken together, these axes define a number of cells or boxes—the number limited only by the imagination and energy of the analyst. The job of program developers or community planners is to enumerate and fill in the missing boxes. If there is no Medicaid-reimbursable social day care in the community, it must be developed; home care services must be reorganized to provide for the non-Medicare client; and so forth.

Similarly, the task of service coordinator, discharge planner, or case manager in this model is to perform an assessment of each client seeking to enter the system in order to determine in precisely which box the client belongs. If the appropriate box does not exist, then the client presumably bounces randomly until he or she ends up in the wrong box. (1987, pp. 6-7)

Vladeck (1987) suggests that we must change these metaphors. Using the metaphor of a root and branch system of a tree would make us more client responsive. The client, perceived as a tree, is supported by the system. Roots reach out in all directions to find the necessary resources to sustain the tree, and branches in the form of client options grow and develop, nurtured by the roots.

The tree metaphor places the service delivery system in support of the client. As client needs are identified, services are developed to meet those needs. As services develop, so do classification schemes. As needs change, the process continues — new and different services are developed. The delivery system, then, evolves as communities change. Often, however, the roots become entangled and there are snarls within the delivery system. Gaining an understanding of the existing root system is a challenge. Social workers, as advocates, can begin reframing the way the hospital is perceived in the long-term delivery system.

On a micro level, ethical dilemmas constantly arise in the course of social work practice. Hospital-based long-term care programs are no exception. Regardless of where the social worker is placed within the hospital system, s/he must constantly advocate for clients and assist in decision-making.

Social workers committed to serving those who cannot pay find that hospitals are not always sensitive to these issues. For example, a social worker in a large metropolitan hospital-based case management program was told by her supervisor that they were raising their fees. For several older clients, this would be an impossibility. The social worker approached the hospital auxiliary to begin a scholarship fund for older persons who needed case management but who had no resources. The social worker's ability to network and to problem solve made the difference between whether clients would be abandoned or would continue to receive service.

As social workers play transitional manager, post acute, and chronic care roles, they often observe former acute care staff having difficulty adjusting. Whereas acute care systems operate in a paternalistic mode, doing for the patient, the intent of long-term care is to rehabilitate. To regain functioning, clients must be allowed to do things for themselves. One social worker attached to a swing-bed unit watched a nurse work with an elderly man. In a caring and loving manner, the nurse did tasks for the man that would take him ten times as long to do. It seemed to be a waste of time for him to spend so much time working on a simple task such as dialing a telephone. The transition between acute care roles and long-term care roles can be traumatic for some staff who are trained to work quickly and efficiently, only to find themselves in long-term care settings in which deliberate, slower actions are required. The social worker who is trained in long-term care services may actually assist others in understanding the diverse needs of long-term care recipients.

A similar example occurred in a metropolitan hospital system that had recently acquired a long-term care facility. To staff this facility, a different medical social worker from the hospital acute care department was assigned to the facility every afternoon on a rotating basis. Although this type schedule might work in an acute care setting in which patients come and go quickly, seeing a new face every day was confusing to and lacked continuity for residents.

Hospital diversification may be used as a strategy to increase visibility and enhance public relations in the community. In these circumstances, social workers are often viewed as marketers. For example, a hospital social worker serving as discharge planner found that several patients needed homemaker services. Fees for homemaker services were highly competitive within the community. The social worker referred discharged patients to a community-based agency that offered services at the most reasonable cost. A supervisor questioned why the social worker would not refer to the hospital-based in-home care program. Potential conflicts of interest are inevitable when large systems deliver diverse services and referrals are made between units.

In summary, health care social workers are performing multiple roles within hospital-based long-term care programs for the elderly.

Regardless of what role is performed, the concept of advocacy for the client undergirds practice. Not only is the practitioner challenged to use more client-sensitive metaphors to reconceptualize the system on a macro level, but s/he is engaged in daily ethical decision-making with and for older clients.

REFERENCES

Abramson, Julie S. (1988). Participation of elderly patients in discharge planning: Is self-determination a reality? *Social Work, 33,* 443-448.

Aiello, Daniel (1988, November). Survey finds diversification growing corporate strategy. *Provider, 14*(11), 24-27.

Balinsky, Warren & Rehman, Sabeeha (1984, Spring). Home health care: A comparative analysis of hospital-based and community-based agency patients. *Home Health Care Services Quarterly, 5*(1), 45-60.

Ballis, Susan (May-June 1985). A case for generic social work in health settings. *Social Work, 30*(3), 209-212.

Bendor, Susan J. (1987). The clinical challenge of hospital-based social work practice. *Social Work in Health Care, 13*(2), 25-34.

Bennett, Clarie Johnson & Grob, Gail Green (1982, Winter). The social worker new to health care: Basic learning tasks. *Social Work in Health Care, 8*(2), 49-64.

Bergstrom, Christine (1979, Summer). The teaching social worker in family medicine: A prototype for the hospital social worker? *Social Work in Health Care, 4*(4), 409-419.

Berkman, Barbara, Kemler, Beth, Marcus, Leonard, & Silverman, Phyllis (1985, Fall). Course content for social work practice in health care. *Journal of Social Work Education, 21*(3), 43-51.

Blumenfield, Susan & Rosenberg, Gary (1988). Towards a network of social health services: Redefining discharge planning and expanding the social work domain. *Social Work in Health Care, 13*(4), 31-48.

Borland, James J. & Strauss, Marc (1982, August). Social work education for health care: A blueprint for action. *Health and Social Work, 7*(3), 224-229.

Bowlyow, Joyce E. (1989, February). Long-term care in small rural hospitals. *The Gerontologist, 29*(1), 81-85.

Bracht, Neil F. (1983, Spring). Preparing new generations of social workers to practice in health settings. *Social Work and Health Care, 8*(3), 29-54.

Capitman, John A., Prottas, Jeffrey, MacAdam, Margaret, Leutz, Walter, Westwater, Don & Yee, Donna L. (1988). A descriptive framework for new hospital roles in geriatric care. *Health Care Financing Review,* Annual Supplement, 17-25.

Carlton, Thomas Owen (1988). Editorial: Out of hospital health care. *Health and Social Work, 13*(1), 5-8.

Coulton, Claudia J., Dunkle, Ruth E., Chow, Julian Chun-Chung, Haug, Marie,

& Bielhaber, David P. (1988, April). Dimensions of post-hospital care decision-making: A factor analytic study. *The Gerontologist, 28*(2), 218-223.

Dubler, Nancy Neveloff (1988, June). Improving the discharge planning process: Distinguishing between coercion and choice. *The Gerontologist, 28*(Suppl), 76-81.

Eisdorfer, Carol & Maddox, George (Eds.) (1988). *The Role of Hospitals in Geriatric Care*. New York: Springer Publishing Company.

Fischer, Lucy Rose & Eustis, Nancy N. (1988). DRGs and family care for the elderly: A case study. *The Gerontologist, 28*(3), 383-389.

Gonyea, Judith G., Seltzer, Gary B., Gerstein, Claire, & Young, Malka (1988, Summer). Acceptance of hospital-based respite care by families and elders. *Health and Social Work, 13*(3), 201-208.

Graves, Edmund J. (1987, July 2). Diagnosis-related groups using data from the national discharge survey: United States, 1985. *Advancedata*, Number 137, U.S. Department of Health and Human Services National Center for Health Statistics.

Kerson, Toba Schwaber (1979, Spring). Sixty years ago: Hospital social work in 1918. *Social Work in Health Care, 4*(3), 331-343.

Lane, Helen J. (1982, August). Toward the preparation of social work specialists in health care. *Health and Social Work, 7*(3), 230-233.

Lawrance, Frances P. (1988). Discharge planning social work focus. In Volland, Patricia J. (Ed.). *Discharge Planning: An Interdisciplinary Approach to Continuity of Care*. Owings Mill, MD: National Health Publishing, pp. 119-152.

Peterson, K. Jean (1987). Changing needs of patients and families in the acute care hospital: Implications for social work practice. *Social Work in Health Care, 13*(2), 1-14.

Prybil, Lawrence D. (1980, Fall). Provision of long-term care services by community hospitals in Virginia. *Hospital and Health Services Administration, 25*(4), 80-102.

Rauch, Julia B. & Schreiber, Hanita (1985, Summer). Discharge planning as a teaching mechanism. *Health and Social Work, 10*(3), 208-216.

Read, William A., & O'Brien, J. L. (1986). *Emerging trends in aging and long-term care services*. Chicago: The Hospital Research and Educational Trust.

Ritvo, Roger A. (1988). Coordinating in-patient and out-patient services: The need for action. *Social Work in Health Care, 13*(1), 39-56.

Rocheleau, Bruce (1983). *Hospitals and Community Oriented Programs for the Elderly*. Ann Arbor, MI: AUPHA Press.

Rubenstein, Laurence Z. (1987, Fall). Innovations in hospital care for elders. *Generations, 12*(1), 65-70.

Simmons, W. June & White, Monika (1988). *Case management and discharge planning: Two different worlds*. In Volland, Patricia J. Discharge Planning: An Interdisciplinary Approach to Continuity of Care, Owings Mill, MD: National Health Publishing, pp. 217-238.

Vladeck, Bruce C. (1988). Hospitals, the elderly, and comprehensive care. In

Eisdorfer, Carl & Maddox, George L. (Eds.). *The Role of Hospitals in Geriatric Care*. New York: Springer Publishing Company, pp. 35-48.

Vladeck, Bruce C. (1987). The continuum of care: Principles and metaphors. In Evanwick, Connie J., and Weiss, Lawrence J. (Eds.). *Managing the Continuum of Care*. Rockville, MD: Aspen Publishers, pp. 3-10.

Williams, Frank G., Netting, F. Ellen, & Hood-Szivek, Pamela (1988, August). Developing swing bed programs in rural Arizona hospitals. *The Gerontologist*, 28(4), 495-498.

Wolkenstein, Alan S. & Laufenburg, Herbert F. (1981, Spring). Teaching the behavioral science component in a family practice residency: Social work role. *Social Work in Health Care*, 6(3), 35-47.

Wolock, Isabel, Schleslinger, Elfriede, Dinerman, Miriam, & Seaton, Richard (1987, Summer). The posthospital needs and care of patients: Implications for discharge planning. *Social Work in Health Care*, 12(4), 61-76.

Utilizing Client Experience in Developing New Service Delivery Models for Care of the Aged

Phyllis H. Mutschler
James J. Callahan, Jr.

SUMMARY. The utilization experience of control group members of the National Long Term Care Demonstration (Channeling) is assumed to represent ordinary use of services by this population. Patterns of utilization over 12 months are examined and the implications of these patterns for design of new service delivery models are explored.

In the late 1950s the National Commission on Chronic Illness issued a report on care of the long term patient. It described how the long duration of the needs of these patients required different approaches from those of the acute patient and called for better and different services, as well as a degree of coordination. The report was oriented toward individual patients and their health concerns. After Medicare and Medicaid became established in the late 1960s, the policy focus shifted, from a focus on the individual patient to reform of the long term care system through changes in financing, reimbursement and organization. This paper will attempt to integrate the experience of long term care clients into designing delivery systems for long term care of the aged.

The human services system affecting older persons grew dramatically with the expansion of federal and state programs of the '60s.

Support for this research was provided by the Farnsworth Trust (State Street Bank and Trust Company Trustee) of The Medical Foundation of Boston, MA.

In the space of a few years, Congress enacted Medicare, Medicaid, the Older Americans Act, the Economic Opportunity Act, and the Model Cities Program, expanded Old Age and Survivors Disability Insurance, and in the early '70s created the Supplemental Security Income Program. Rapid growth occurred in all these programs, particularly for in-home and community services, as will be described below.

Despite, or perhaps as part of, this impressive growth in the domain of long-term care, a number of problems emerged. For the past 20 years they have been recited as a virtual litany by policymakers. Callahan and Wallack (1981) listed the problems as:

a. persistence of unmet needs in the population
b. bias towards institutionalization
c. low levels of the quality of care produced
d. geographical inequity and maldistribution of benefits
e. excessive burdens placed on families
f. rapidly rising public and private expenditures
g. fragmentation among services and financing
h. lack of case management functions

To begin to confront these problems, a series of long-term care demonstration projects were launched in the mid-1970s with a few continuing to the present time.

While not all of the research is complete on all of the projects, a number of important syntheses of the results of the demonstrations and studies have been published. The Health Care Financing Administration (HCFA) devoted its 1988 Annual Supplement of the Health Care Financing Review to the results of research of post-acute and long-term care. The National Governors' Association (1988) reviewed the development of community care systems in six states as part of its effort to reform long-term care.

Kane and Kane (1987) reviewed over 200 studies and reports to answer the questions: "What have several decades of research and demonstration taught us that could help us decide how to spend the next dollar for long-term care? How might each community's particular history and characteristics affect such decisions?" (p. 9).

Weissert, Cready and Pawelak examined over 700 citations on

the results of home and community care studies conducted over the past 25 years. They examined: "the extent to which patients served in the studies reviewed were at risk of using a nursing home or hospital; how much their institutional care use was reduced by using home and community care; how much outpatient care use was reduced by home and community care use; what the cost of new services was; savings or losses resulting from changes in use of existing and new services; and, effects on various domains of health status.

The results of these analyses generally show a failure to achieve the high hopes they promised for resolving the problems of the long-term care system. Kane and Kane (1987) note that ". . . some positive results have been associated with some of the demonstrations. Taken together, however, the results on mortality and quality of life are, at best, ambiguous, and the results on the use of and cost of other services is discouraging" (p. 336). Kemper and Applebaum (1987), who conducted a review of 16 major projects concluded:

> What the demonstrations have shown is that expanding publicly funded case management and community care does not reduce aggregate costs, and is likely to increase them — at least in the current long-term care service environment, which already provides some community care under Medicare, Medicaid, and other public programs. Small reductions in nursing home costs for some are more than offset by the increased costs of providing expanded community services to others who, even without expanded services, would not enter nursing homes.

Although the demonstrations showed little impact on the rates of institutionalization, an anticipated expansion in the use of nursing homes failed to occur. Consider the following facts. In 1977, the Congressional Budget Office (1977) estimated that the number of persons in nursing homes would increase from about 1.3 million in 1977 to 2.2 million in 1985. By 1985, however, only 1.5 million persons were residing in nursing homes — an increase of only 200,000, rather than the 900,000 increase that had been expected;

nearly three-quarters of a million fewer people were in nursing homes.[1] Moreover, in 1977, there were 59.7 beds per thousand elders; seven years later, in 1985, this number dropped to 56.9 beds per thousand elders. At the same time, for every thousand persons over 65, the number of residents in nursing homes dropped from 47.9 to 46. Occupancy of nursing homes rose from 89 to 91.6 percent and the population became older and more disabled (NCHS, 1987). If the 1977 estimate had been correct, then families and communities or alternate institutions (e.g., hospitals, specialized residences) have absorbed some 800,000 expected nursing home admissions.

A number of factors are responsible for the lack of growth of the institutional population: the certificate of need requirements enacted in many states, the elimination of the "step up in value" provisions of rate setting formulas, and the high interest rates during the late 1970s restrained the supply of beds. Due to a number of factors, consumer demand also declined. The proportion of individuals "inappropriately placed" in nursing homes, which had ranged from anywhere from 40-70 percent of the residents, diminished. Housing choices for older persons expanded. And, due to the cost of living adjustments in social security and SSI, older persons' incomes improved relative to the general population.

However, perhaps the most important factor accounting for communities' capacity to absorb the predicted institutional population was the dramatic growth in home care reflected both in home health expenditures under Medicare and Medicaid, and by expansion in the number of certified home health agencies. For example, between 1973 and 1985 the annual growth rate in home health expenditures under Medicare was 26.1 percent per year. In 1973, home health expenditures accounted for only 1 percent of the total Medicare budget and by 1985 that reached 3.1 percent. Medicaid increased even more dramatically during this time: home health expenditures grew at an annual rate of 38.5 percent. In 1973 home

---

1. While there are some slight differences between the 1977 definitions of nursing homes and that of the 1985 National Nursing Home Survey, they are not significant enough to affect the discrepancy.

health expenditures were only .3 percent of Medicaid but by 1985 they reached 3 percent. Both the number of persons served and the numbers of visits per person grew as well. For every thousand persons over 65, in 1974, Medicare provided home care to about 17 persons; but by 1985 home care services reached nearly 56 persons per thousand. Visits per persons also increased from 20.6 in 1974 to 27.3 in 1983 (Bishop and Stassen, 1985).

This increased utilization generated an expansion in the number of certified home health agencies. They increased by 65 percent from 2,212 in 1972 to reach 3,639 in 1982. Then, in the brief four year period 1982 to 1986, there was another increase of about 65 percent with the number of home health agencies growing from 3,639 to 6,012 (*Home Health Line*, 1988).[2]

The ambiguous results of the research and demonstration projects, however, have not deterred the search for policy solutions. Efforts continue to be made in both private and public sectors and at both the Federal and State levels to improve the financing and organization of long-term care services. These strategies have been described and evaluated by Rivlin and Wiener (1988) in a book published recently by the Brookings Institute. Within the private sector they review: private long-term care insurance, continuing care retirement communities, the social/health maintenance organization, individual medical accounts, home equity conversion, and selected changes in the delivery system. On the public side, they discuss block grants, a liberalized Medicaid program, public long-term care insurance, family responsibility, public support for unpaid caregivers and public expansion of home care. For each of these approaches, they project future costs and utilization, showing who would benefit most by a particular reform and what would be the impact on public expenditures.

Attempts at reform in the public sector are embodied in numerous legislative bills that have been introduced in Congress including those of Senators Kennedy, Mitchell, Melcher and Representatives Waxman, Stark and the late Claude Pepper. However, the one ma-

---

2. It now appears, however, that the expansion in this market is slowing down as Medicare cuts back on reimbursement so that the number of visits per person is beginning to fall.

jor piece of legislation that was passed in 1988—the Medicare Catastrophic Act—has received such negative reaction that other legislative remedies may be derailed.

Successful implementation of any of these initiatives will need to address the real or apparent contradiction between, on the one hand, the trends observed over time in nursing home placements and home care service utilization and, on the other, the results of the individual demonstration programs that did not show large tradeoffs between community and institutional services. If reform of long-term care is to be effective, it must be informed by an understanding of client utilization careers. System design cannot proceed successfully without a longitudinal view of service use and transitions from one set of services to another. To date, little research has been undertaken that allows for detailed examination of elders' patterns of service of utilization over time. This paper attempts to add to the research by examining the experience of elders in the control group of the National Long Term Care Demonstration known as Channeling to try to understand how older persons used the existing systems of services that were available in the community.

The Channeling Demonstration took place in 10 communities and tested a basic case management model and a case management model where the case managers had some control of funding. The demonstration had both an experimental group and a control group. The control group did not receive the case management intervention, but their utilization of services was carefully tracked and documented. This study assumes that the patterns of utilization of the control group represent the way older persons would have used those services if there had been no channeling intervention.[3] In other words, the control group's experience is a natural experiment representing usual and ordinary patterns of service use in the target communities. As such, it provides an opportunity to examine some of the assumptions about utilization that underlie current policy proposals.

This paper examines the types of services used, the consistency in utilization over a 12 month period, and the extent of case man-

---

3. While the survey process itself may have had some influence on client behavior, we do not consider this a serious problem.

agement. It looks also at the association of formal service use with elders: health status or disability; informal support system; and/or sociodemographic characteristics (race, age, sex, education, financial status, household composition, and urban-rural residence).

DATA SOURCE AND SAMPLE

The data allowing for this detailed examination were contained in four of the fourteen channeling demonstration public use analysis files. These files provided elders' responses to survey questions at baseline and follow-up interviews at six and twelve months, and from claims data. Survey items focused on (1) formal services provided by community agencies, (2) informal care, and (3) medical and long-term care services. Of the 2173 elders who comprised the control group at baseline, 327 had died by the six month follow-up interviews, and another 234 had died by the end of a year; another 111 individuals were missing at both six and 12 months follow-up interviews.

A PROFILE OF THE CONTROL GROUP

As can be seen in Table 1, the demographic characteristics of the control group, their functional limitations, and informal care arrangements are typical of frail elders in many other studies. Most sample members (45%) were between 75 and 84 years of age, but one in ten was 90 years or older, and one in eight was less than 70 years of age. The typical respondent was a widowed white woman, in poor health, who had only an elementary school education, and who lived in an urban area. However, while over half the sample lived in a large city, nearly one in twenty lived in a small city, and another one in eight resided in a rural area or suburban setting. Half the sample had monthly incomes below $447, while the average annual income was $6,408.

Most sample members were severely impaired in performing both activities of daily living (ADLs) and instrumental activities of daily living (IADLs). Only one in twenty had mild limitations in dressing, eating, bathing, getting out of bed, or using the toilet, whereas 56 percent had severe or extremely severe difficulties in

TABLE 1

BACKGROUND CHARACTERISTICS OF SAMPLE POPULATION
(N=2173)[a]

Age	
64-69	12%
70-74	17%
75-79	22%
80-84	23%
85-89	17%
90+	10%
Sex	
Female	72%
Male	28%
Race	
White and Others	75%
Black	22%
Hispanic	3%
Marital Status[b]	
Currently Married	31%
Widowed	56%
Divorced	4%
Separated	2%
Never Married	7%

56

Educational Level
Elementary School or Less | 57%
High School | 33%
Some College | 11%

Type of Community
Large City. 2.500.000 | 47%
Suburb of Large City | 15%
Medium Sized City. 50.000 | 10%
Suburb of Medium Sized City | 10%
Small City | 5%
Small Town or Rural | 13%

Living Arrangements
Lives with Spouse | 30%
Lives :with Child | 22%
Lives with Others | 11%
Lives Alone:
With Informal Support | 29%
Without Informal Support | 8%

Income
Mean Monthly Income in 1982 | $534.00
Median Monthly Income in 1982 | $446.00

Health Status
Excellent | 2%
Good | 16%
Fair | 29%
Poor | 53%

57

TABLE 1 (continued)

Functional Dependency
1. Dependent in Activities in Daily Living (ADLs)
    Mild or No Impairment   20%
    Moderate Impairment   24%
    Severe Impairment   34%
    Extreme Impairment   22%

2. Dependent in Instrumental Activities of Daily Living (IADLs)[c]
    Mild Impairment   5%
    Moderate Impairment   25%
    Severe Impairment   30%
    Extreme Impairment   40%

Number of Days in Bed: Two Months Prior to Baseline
Mean Monthly Number of Days   19
Median Monthly Number of Days   6

Use of Nursing Homes & Hospitals: Two Months Prior to Baseline
1. Nursing Homes
    Mean Monthly Number of Days   28
    Median Monthly Number of Days   23

2. Hospitalization
    Mean Monthly Number of Days   19
    Median Monthly Number of Days   14

58

In Nursing Home at
  6 Months 7%
  12 Months 10%
  6 and 12 Months 16%

Mortality
  Dead at 6 Months 15%
  Dead at 12 Months[d] ... 26%

----

a   Percentages greater of less than 100% reflect rounding.
b   Based on 2169 elders.
c   Based on 2068 elders.
d   Percentage of sample members dead at 12 months includes sample members who
    had died at 6 months. Of 1355 people alive at 6 months. 234 (17%) died by
    12 months.

performing these tasks. Even higher proportions (70%) of elders had great difficulty shopping, preparing meals, telephoning, managing money or doing light housework. Given such impairments, it is not at all surprising that less than one in twenty rated their health as good or excellent, while 53 percent said they were in poor health. Yet, sample members made modest use of hospitals (14 days per year) and nursing homes (23 days per year).

UTILIZATION OF FORMAL SERVICES

The analysis focused on the use of formal services reported by the control group at baseline, six and twelve months. Formal services were defined as those tasks and services performed by persons employed by health and social service agencies as well as by other types of paid helpers who provided services in the elder's home. Sixteen individual services were grouped into four categories: medical services, home delivered services, community-based services, and case management.

Medical services included physician visits, nursing home episodes and hospital admissions. *Home delivered services* included meal preparation by a formal provider, whether living in the household or visiting it; meals delivered to the home; help with housework such as laundry, shopping or chores; personal care; and, medical treatments provided at home by physical, occupational, and speech therapists; and home health aide services. These were individualized and scheduled for particular clients in their own homes. *Community-based services* were not available at home but were provided by agencies in the community such as: social or recreational programs; day health programs; meals at Senior Centers; transportation; and counseling or mental health services. *Case management services* were defined as those services that provide initial client needs assessment, care planning, making arrangements for services, and ongoing monitoring of client needs. These services were provided by a variety of agencies, including: special channeling-like programs, state-funded home care services, mental health and community counseling agencies, integrated social service agencies, and home health agencies. They may have been a separate service or a component of another service.

As shown in Table 2, medical services were used by the largest number — nearly 100 percent — of elders, followed by in-home services. Given the sample's level of impairment in ADLs and IADLs, use of in-home and medical services is consistent with the findings in other studies.

Although the proportions of elders using in-home or medical services remained relatively stable over the twelve months, the proportion of elders using community services dropped dramatically. This decrease is primarily a consequence of increasing frailty among surviving sample members.[4]

PATTERNS OF SERVICE USE

Simply knowing what services older persons use is inadequate for designing new models. It is important to know how combinations of services are used and if any patterns result. The four service categories, therefore, were cross-classified to produce sixteen patterns of use that would be possible at each point in time — baseline, 6 and 12 months. The distribution of the sample across these sixteen patterns is shown in Table 3.

At Baseline

At the baseline interview, only one out of every 25 elders said they used no services at all, and only one individual listed case management as the sole service used. Relatively few individuals used community services either alone (1 percent) or in combination with one other type of service; although 8 percent used both community and medical services and another 6 percent used community, in-home and medical services without benefit of case management. Only 4 percent used all four types of services.

On the other hand, medical services, alone or in combination with other services, were widely used. Twenty-three percent of the sample used medical services only, and another 28 percent used

---

4. Certain counseling services were excluded from the definition of community services at six and twelve months; this may account for a very small amount of this decreased utilization of community services. However, most studies of elders' service use show that fewer than five percent utilize counselling services.

TABLE 2

UTILIZATION OF FORMAL SERVICES
AT BASELINE, SIX AND TWELVE MONTHS

Type of Service	Percent Received Service at:		
	Baseline N=2173	Six Months N=1846	Twelve Months N=1386
Home Services	63%	49%	54%
Community-based Services	20%	6%	8%
Case Management	27%	35%	32%
Medical Services	90%	99%	91%

TABLE 3

SERVICE UTILIZATION PATTERN AT BASELINE, SIX AND TWELVE MONTHS

	Baseline (N=2173)	Six Mos. (N=2173)	Twelve Mos. (N=2173)
No Services	3.9%	3.9%	4.8%
Case Mgt. Only	.0%	.7%	.5%
Case Mgt. & Medical Only	.1%	5.8%	2.7%
Case Mgt.. Community. Medical	.3%	.3%	.3%
All Services	4.1%	2.0%	1.6%
Only Home Services	2.3%	3.3%	3.4%
Community and Home Only	.3%	.2%	.4%
Medical and Home Only	28.1%	13.8%	11.4%
Case Mgt.. Home. Medical	20.3%	17.3%	10.9%

TABLE 3 (continued)

Medical Services Only	23.2%	19.1%	16.4%
Medical and Community Only	8.4%	1.1%	.8%
All. But No Case Mgt.	5.9%	1.6%	1.1%
Case Mgt. & Community Only	.0%	.3%	.1%
Community Only	1.0%	.2%	.3%
Case Mgt. & Home Only	1.7%	3.1%	3.5%
Case Mgt.. Home. Community	.3%	.1%	.2%
Dead by Six or Twelve Month Interview	.0%	15.0%	25.8%
Unknown at Six or Twelve Month Interview	.0%	12.1%	16.1%
TOTAL	100.0%	100.0%	100.0%

medical services along with paid in-home services. One out of every five elders received medical services combined with case management and in-home services. Yet, only 2 percent used in-home paid help without receiving other services, and another 2 percent combined case management with in-home services, but did not receive medical care.

At Six Months

By six months (Table 4), 15 percent of the elders had died, and another 12 percent had been lost to follow up. Those who remained, however, exhibited a pattern of service use that was very close to that reported at baseline interviews. Slightly more than a quarter of those who were surveyed at six months used medical services only, and nearly one in five used medical and paid in-home help; nearly a quarter received case management along with medical and in-home services.

Conversely, nearly one in twenty elders used no services at all, and — as was true at baseline — very few used community services alone (4 percent) or in combination with other types of service. Only 35 elders, compared with 129 elders at baseline, used a combination of community, medical and in-home services, but did not receive case management. The number of individuals receiving a combination of case management and in-home services, though small, nearly doubled between baseline and 6 months, from 37 to 67 elders.

At Twelve Months

By the time of the 12 month follow-up interviews (Table 5), more than one-third of the sample had been lost: 26 percent were dead and another 12 percent were missing. Another 5 percent who had been missing at six months were interviewed at twelve months, but their responses are not used in this analysis. Of the 1264 elders who remain, the largest number, 28 percent, were using only medical services, although nearly one-fifth received medical services and services provided in the home by paid helpers. Approximately another fifth received medical and in-home services along with case management. Very few elders (3 percent) received all four types of

TABLE 4

PATTERNS OF CHANGE IN SERVICE UTILIZATION

	ALIVE & KNOWN AT 12 MONTHS (N=1264)[a]
Same Pattern Baseline 6 and 12 months	13.2%
Change Pattern Between 6 and 12 months only	13.0%
Change Pattern Between Baseline & 6 months But Remain in Same Pattern Between 6 and 12 months	29.4%
Change Between Baseline and 6 months But Change Back in Baseline Pattern at 12 months	10.8%

Change Between Baseline and 6 months
And Again between 6 and 12 months   33.6%

---

a Of 2173 Elders at Baseline.

Died by 6 months   15.0%
Died between 6 and 12 months   10.8%

No change baseline to 6 months   (N=45)   19%
Change between baseline & 6 mos. (N=189)   81%

Unknown Status   5.1%

TABLE 5

TRANSITIONS BETWEEN SERVICE PATTERNS AT SIX AND TWELVE MONTHS
FOR ELDERS WHO USED ONLY MEDICAL SERVICES AT BASELINE

Of 504 Who Used Only Medical Services at Baseline

26.6% Died at 6 Months (N=134)

7.1% Used No Services at 6 Months (N=36)

Died	N=8	(22.2%)
Used No Services	N=15	(41.7%)
Case Mgt. W/ or W/O Other Services	N=1	(2.8%)
Services Without Case Management	N=4	(11.1%)
Case Mgt., Home & Medical Services	N=1	(2.8%)
Medical and In-Home Services Only	N=2	(5.6%)
Medical Services Only	N=5	(13.9%)

10.5% Used Case Mgt. W/ or W/O Other Services[a] at 6 Months (N=53)

Died	N=13	(24.5%)
Used No Services	N=3	(5.7%)
Case Mgt. W/ or W/O Other Services	N=5	(9.4%)
Services Without Case Management	N=7	(13.4%)
Case Mgt., Home & Medical Services	N=5	(9.4%)
Medical and In-Home Services Only	N=2	(3.8%)
Medical Services Only	N=18	(34.0%)

4% Used Some Services Without Case Mgt. at 6 Months (N=20)

Died	N=1	(5.8%)
Used No Services	N=2	(10.0%)
Case Mgt. W/ or W/O Other Services	N=6	(30.0%)
Services Without Case Management	N=4	(20.0%)
Case Mgt., Home & Medical Services	N=4	(20.0%)
Medical and In-Home Services Only	N=1	(5.0%)
Medical Services Only	N=2	(10.0%)

Of 504 Who
Used Only Medical
Services at
Baseline

10.3% Used Only Medical & In-Home Services at 6 Months (N=52)

Category	N	%
Died	N=12	(23.1%)
Used No Services	N=1	(1.9%)
Case Mgt. W/ or W/O Other Services	N=2	(3.8%)
Services Without Case Management	N=4	(7.7%)
Case Mgt.. Home & Medical Services	N=7	(13.5%)
Medical and In-Home Services Only	N=13	(25.0%)
Medical SErvices Only	N=13	(25.0%)

10.3% Used Case Mgt.. Home & Medical Services at 6 Months (N=52)

Category	N	%
Died	N=12	(23.1%)
Used No Services	N=1	(1.9%)
Case Mgt. W/ or W/O Other Services	N=7	(13.5%)
Services Without Case Management	N=4	(7.7%)
Case Mgt.. Home & Medical Services	N=14	(26.9%)
Medical and In-Home Services Only	N=10	(19.2%)
Medical Services Only	N=4	(7.7%)

31.2% Used Only Medical Services at 6 Months (N=157)

Category	N	%
Died	N=33	(21.0%)
Used No Services	N=17	(10.8%)
Case Mgt. W/ or W/O Other Services	N=9	(5.7%)
Services Without Case Management	N=7	(4.5%)
Case Mgt.. Home & Medical Services	N=6	(3.8%)
Medical and In-Home Services Only	N=14	(8.9%)
Medical Services Only	N=71	(45.2%)

----

a Services combined with Case Management include either Community, Medical, Home, or all three; Community and Home or Community and Medical.

b Home Services Only, Community Services Only, Medical and Community, Home and Community.

services and services provided in the home by paid helpers. Approximately another fifth received medical and in-home services along with case management. Very few elders (3 percent) received all four types of service and one in twelve received no services at all — an increase of three percentage points over the six month survey.

CHANGES IN PATTERNS OF SERVICE

It is tempting to assume, since the most prevalent patterns of service remain the same from baseline through the twelve month survey, that elders select a group of services to suit their needs and continue to use them over time. Quite the contrary is true. As shown in Table 4, only 13 percent of elders used the same mix of services at six and twelve months that they had reported at baseline. The largest proportion of elders — more than one-third — received a different mix of services at baseline, six and twelve months. Another 11 percent changed their utilization pattern between baseline and six months, and again between six months and one year, but the "twelve month" pattern was the same as that reported during baseline interviews. Nearly three in ten elders used a different pattern of services at six months than they had reported at baseline, but the "six month" pattern persisted between the six month and one year follow-up interviews. We see from these statistics that certain groupings of services may enjoy heavy use at all times, but individual elders shift their pattern of use over the one year period. Thus, the stability of the service system has masked the dynamic quality of elders' service use.

SERVICE CAREERS

How do elders who began with a particular mix of services move into other services? Were they adding services over time, or shifting among service types? To trace the elders' service "careers" over the year between baseline, six and twelve months, we created a smaller number of categories. By combining those service patterns that were less prevalent, six patterns of service utilization were established:

1. No Services.
2. Case Management With or Without Other Services.
3. Some Services But No Case Management.
4. Case Management, In-Home and Medical Services.
5. Medical and In-Home Services Only.
6. Medical Services Only.

Certain groups of services in which case management is a component were combined into one category, titled "Case Management With or Without Other Services." This category contains case management alone, or together with any services except the combination of in-home and medical services. The other cluster of service patterns that were less prevalent included services that were used without any case management intervention. These included: in-home services only, community services only, medical and community services, or in-home and community services.

TRANSITIONS IN SERVICE UTILIZATION PATTERNS

Greater frailty characterized those using medical care alone or in combination with in-home or case management services at baseline. Consequently, we expected that these groups would be likely to maintain a stable mix of services or to add services over time to compensate for increased impairments. We were surprised to find, however, that even these elders shifted the kinds of services they used. To illustrate such transitions, the service utilization "careers" of those 504 elders who, at baseline, had used medical services are presented in Table 5. Only 31 percent of those who had used medical services at baseline persisted in this pattern at six months. One-tenth added in-home services at six months and another tenth added both in-home and case management services to their medical service use. On the other hand, 7 percent ceased using any services by six months, while another 15 percent selected an alternative cluster of services.

Of those who added in-home services to medical services by the six month survey, one-quarter continued to receive these services, but one in four dropped the in-home services again between six and twelve months. More than one-quarter of elders who had added both in-home and case management to medical services at six months maintained that package of services at twelve months; however, nearly one in five continued to receive in-home services but dropped case management from the services they received. What emerges from following these utilization "careers" is that elders change the mix of services they use. Some may find a package of service that will help them maintain a desired level of functioning, and thus will continue to use these services over time. More often, however, elders do not persist in the use of a particular service mix, but instead shift their use to reflect their changing circumstances.

There may be some objection that the amount of change observed over the 12 months is the result of looking at too detailed a level of services that might be substituted for each other. The dynamic pattern holds up, however, when the data are analyzed for only one category; for example, in-home services. Sixty-three percent of the control group used such services at baseline. By six months, however, only half of the users continued to use these services, while 27 percent of those without home services at baseline received them. Of this latter group, however, only 57 percent still had in-home services by twelve months.

CONSIDERATIONS FOR DEVELOPING
NEW MODELS OF CARE

The findings of this study have implications for the design of new models of care. First, the data show that older persons and their caretakers make heavy use of formal services as elders become more disabled. The use of formal services exists side by side with informal care. This reinforces findings beginning with the 1977 Cleveland GAO study up to the National Long Term Care Survey of 1982 and 1984. Since this is an existing pattern, one needs to ask to what extent and under what conditions should new models attempt to change this pattern. Should families and individuals be encouraged to take responsibility and control for finding and utilizing their own services as many now do? Should a major information program be developed so that people know where to turn and when? What impact might a mandated case management and assessment program for access to long term care benefits have on this existing pattern of utilization? Would access decrease? Would the case management/assessment function become overwhelmed by the dynamics of the system? Some thought needs to be given to this before one creates, by legislation or administrative organization, single points of assessment and eligibility within a functioning system.

Second, the nearly universal use of medical services by older persons points out the importance of models that link supportive services to this source. Even if medical services are nothing more than "a watering hole," to those who need supportive services, the linkages are important. It is likely, however, that a strategy more than a watering hole approach is needed to integrate better the medical and social services. This finding causes some problems for a purely social model of supportive services. While it is important to maintain the autonomy of supportive services so that they don't become "medicalized," it will be important to design appropriate arrangements to build on the relationship that most frail older persons have with the medical sector.

Third, case management needs to be reviewed as a strategy for meeting the long term care needs of older persons. The findings of this study show that many persons apparently are able to get along without case management and indicate further that many case coordination functions are carried out by individual providers while serving their patients, clients or customers. This is not to say that case management should not be offered, but rather the type, purpose and conditions of case management must be clearly specified.

Fourth, new models must recognize the dynamic nature of the system. Studies by Branch (1977) in Massachusetts show the dynamic change in needs of older persons. There was no inevitable downward trajectory for persons with functional disabilities. This has been verified recently by Manton (1988) and, in the case of nursing home residents, by Shapiro and Tate (1987). The dynamic nature of the system has implications for training of staff who should be taught to expect improvement and renewed independence as well as continued dependence. It points to the need also for good communication between and among families, clients and providers so that changes in status can be acknowledged and appropriate change in service plans take place. Most importantly, it underscores the need for flexible organizational models to handle the changing demands that characterize elders' use of services.

This analysis has shown that the world of long term care is more complicated than simple assumptions would lead one to believe. The conventional wisdom around long term care should be modified by this analysis and others that are coming from the research community. The control group experience of the Channeling Demonstration reveals that within the existing service system elders and service providers together are able to meet needs and satisfy elders' demands with consequences that are no worse in terms of mortality, morbidity, and institutional utilization than a system into which a well designed and funded case management system had been inserted. It is time to learn more about how the present system functions before extensive investments are made in "innovative" ways of improving.

REFERENCES

Bishop, Christine and Stassen, M. (1985). "Prospective reimbursement for home health care." *Pride Institute Journal*, 5, 1, Winter, 17-27.

Branch, L. (1977). *Understanding the health and social service needs of people over age 65*. Cambridge, MA: Center for Living Research, University of Mass. and the Joint Center for Urban Studies of M.I.T. and Harvard University.

Callahan, J. and Wallack, S. (1981). *Reforming the long term care system*. Lexington, MA: Lexington Press.

Congressional Budget Office. (1977). "Long Term Care for the Elderly and Disabled." Washington, D.C.: Congressional Budget Office.

Health Care Financing Review, 1988 Annual Supplement.

Home Health Line. (1988). XIII, May 16, 186.

Kane, R. and Kane, R. (1987). *Long Term Care*. New York: Spring Publishing Co.

Kemper, P. and Applebaum, R. (1987). "A systematic comparison of community care demonstrations," SR #45, Institute for Research on Poverty, Special Report Series, University of Wisconsin-Madison.

Manton, K. (1988). "A longitudinal study of functional change and mortality in the United States." *Journal of Gerontology*, 43, S153-S161.

National Center for Health Statistics. (1987). "Advancedata," 131, March, 27.

Rivilin, A. and Wiener, J. (1988). "Caring for the Disabled Elderly." Washington, D.C.: The Brookings Institution.

Shapiro, Evelyn and Tate, R. (1988). "Who is Really at Risk of Institutionalization?" *The Gerontologist*, 28, 2.

Weissert, W., Cready, C. and Pawelak, J. (1988). "The Past and Future of Community-based Long-Term Care." The Millbank Quarterly, 66, 2.

Models of Intensive Case Management

Gerald M. Eggert
Bruce Friedman
James G. Zimmer

SUMMARY. This article reviews three models of intensive case management developed and tested in Monroe County (Rochester), New York: the Centralized Individual model, the Neighborhood Team, and the Home Health Care Team. The three models are described and contrasted, and the role of the social worker in each is discussed. The models differed especially regarding client assessment and reassessment, direct service provision, and crisis intervention. The cost-effectiveness of the two Team models is highlighted, particularly for dementia and terminal patients. We conclude with a discussion of the relationship between different levels of case management intensity and optimal targeting.

Since case management first evolved for arrangement and coordination of health and social services, a number of different models have been developed. Various demonstration programs and studies conducted over the past fifteen to twenty years have shown the importance of "targeting" interventions to specific types of patients. In this paper we review three models of "intensive" long term care case management that have been developed in Monroe County (Rochester), New York. We conclude with a discussion of lessons

The ACCESS Case Management study was supported by Grants 7794 and 9500 from the Robert Wood Johnson Foundation. The Home Health Care Team study was supported by Grant HS03030 of the National Center for Health Services Research.

The authors wish to express their gratitude to Mary Thompson, Nancy Zaenglein, and Liz Nally for their generous help in reviewing and commenting on earlier drafts of this article.

we have learned about case management, including the applicability of specific case management approaches for different types of cases.

CASE MANAGEMENT

Beginning at least as early as the Worcester Home Care experiment in 1973, case management has been used for the assessment, care plan development, coordination, and arrangement of home and community-based services for long term care patients. Starting with the ACCESS and Georgia Alternative Health Services demonstration programs in 1977, case management has also been utilized to control the amounts of services delivered in order to minimize long term care expenditures. Of the sixteen community care demonstrations that operated under Medicaid and/or Medicare waivers between 1973 and 1984, only one, the National Center for Health Services Research Day Care/Homemaker Experiment, did not include case management (Kemper, Applebaum, and Harrigan, 1987).

Most of the demonstrations used case managers who were individually responsible for a number of cases. Four programs (Triage, Project OPEN, the Multipurpose Senior Services Project, and South Carolina Community Long Term Care) utilized teams of professionals from different disciplines, particularly nursing and social work, to conduct case management (Kemper, Applebaum, and Harrigan, 1987). From 1983 to 1985, both an individual and a team approach were employed at ACCESS.

Twelve of the 19 "most rigorous and generalizable" in-home and community-based care demonstrations and studies for which "critical" health care expenditure data were available included case management (Weissert, Matthews Cready, and Pawelak, 1988). Only four of these 12 were cost-effective. Importantly, however, with one exception that came close (the Channeling Basic Model), none of them isolated case management as the only intervention since additional services were always provided along with case management.

COORDINATION AND INTEGRATION SCHEMES

Case management can best be examined as one component of a community-wide system designed to provide optimal screening, assessment, consultation, management, and service delivery for long term care patients. One of us (Zimmer, 1987) previously created a scheme that shows an optimal system both for persons residing in the community at the time of identification and for those hospitalized when they are identified. This scheme is presented in Figure 1.

Elements of this system have been successfully developed and used, usually as demonstration programs and studies, for substantial periods of time in Monroe County (Rochester), New York (examples include Barker, Williams, Zimmer, Van Buren, Vincent, and Pickrel, 1985; Williams, Williams, Zimmer, Hall, and Podgorski, 1987). Unfortunately, because they were demonstration projects or studies, not all have been continued despite their proven effectiveness. One of the elements of the system is "Intensive Case Management." Three models of "Intensive Case Management" have been tested in Monroe County: The Centralized Individual model, the Neighborhood Case Management Team, and the physician-led Home Health Care Team. These three models are reviewed in this paper.

TARGETING

Most of the studies and demonstration programs whose main purpose was to substitute community-based services and/or home care for institutional care (mostly nursing home care but sometimes hospital care, as well) during the past thirty years cost more than they saved. Of the 19 "most rigorous and generalizable" studies for which "critical" health care expenditure data were available, only seven were cost-effective (Weissert, Matthews Cready, and Pawelak, 1988).

Failure to achieve cost savings has been partially due to poor "targeting," that is, inadequate identification of patients for whom a particular intervention is expected to be cost-effective. The criteria that were expected to identify patients at high risk of nursing home use in fact almost always resulted in the enrollment of low users. In only three of the 22 "most rigorous and generalizable" studies for which data were available did more than one-third of the control group use a nursing home in the twelve months after entering the study (Weissert, Matthews Cready, and Pawelak, 1988).

In Monroe County, the precursors to the recognition of the targeting issue date back to the 1950s when the Monroe County Chronic Illness Committee found many patients in inappropriate settings, for example, long term care patients residing in hospitals rather than in nursing homes (Wenkert and Terris, 1960). In the 1960s the Health Care of Aged Study concluded that 41% of elderly persons receiving health care services were at an inappropriate level of care (University of Rochester, 1968; Wenkert, Hill, and Berg, 1969). The Health Care of Aged Study led directly to the establishment of an Evaluation-Placement Unit at Monroe Community Hospital. This Unit was created to conduct comprehensive assessments of patients who were believed to require admission to long term institutional care. Nearly 85% of patients assessed in the Evaluation-Placement Unit were appropriately placed, a 20-30% improvement over previous Monroe County studies (Williams, Hill, Fairbank, and Knox, 1973). The Evaluation-Placement Unit therefore resulted in better matching of patients with treatment settings.

The importance of matching patients to interventions, i.e., targeting, was thus recognized early in Monroe County. This sensitization of principal actors in the local health care system to the importance of targeting was instrumental in deliberately designing each of two new interventions to serve a specific type of patient. These interventions were the Monroe County Long Term Care Program and the Home Health Care Team. The Monroe County Long Term Care Program, better known as ACCESS, initially targeted patients at the skilled or intermediate levels of care (i.e., the patient would be in a skilled nursing facility or intermediate care facility if institutionalized). The Home Health Care Team was designed to serve chronically and terminally ill homebound elderly persons.

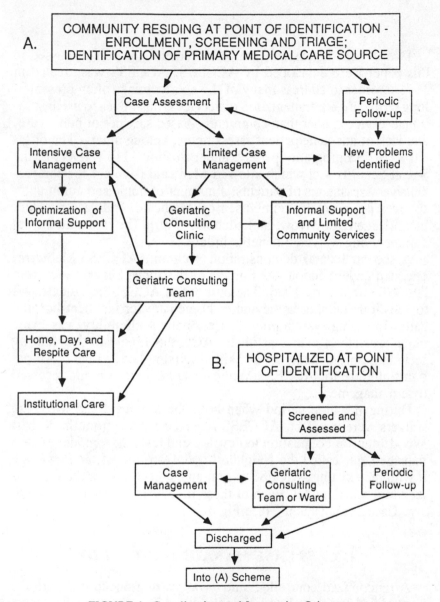

FIGURE 1. Coordination and Integration Schemes

ACCESS

Two of the "Intensive Case Management" models discussed in this paper were developed by ACCESS. ACCESS was created in 1975 in order to address many of the shortcomings often present in long term care — fragmentation of services, incentives to use institutional services rather than community-based services or home care, and lack of adequate patient assessments, among others. The original ACCESS program operated under Section 1115 waivers of the Social Security Act which allowed Medicaid payment for comprehensive assessments of patients, a number of home and community services not normally reimbursed by Medicaid, and case management (Eggert, Bowlyow, and Nichols, 1980). The first patients began receiving waivered benefits in late 1977.

A second federal demonstration program, ACCESS:Medicare, operated under Section 222 waivers of the Social Security Act from late 1982 until early 1986. The purpose of ACCESS:Medicare was to substitute nursing home and/or home care for inpatient hospital care. Targeting was improved (i.e., patient eligibility was made more restrictive) over that of the ACCESS Medicaid program by including only patients at the skilled nursing level of care. All patients eligible for ACCESS:Medicare home care benefits received case management.

During the time period when both the Medicaid and Medicare waivers were in effect, ACCESS received a grant from the Robert Wood Johnson Foundation to develop and test a new model of case management, called the Neighborhood Team model, and compare it with the existing ACCESS case management model, the Centralized Individual model. Each of these models is a variant of "Intensive Case Management" (see Figure 1).

ACCESS CASE MANAGEMENT STUDY

A randomized controlled study was carried out to compare the Centralized Individual and Neighborhood Team case management models (Eggert, Zimmer, Hall, and Friedman, 1989). Between May 1983 and June 1985, ACCESS patients living at home in the northeast quadrant of Rochester, New York were randomized into a treatment or a control group. All patients were assessed as requiring the skilled nursing level of care and were eligible through waivers for payment by Medicare and/or Medicaid of home, community-based, or nursing home services not normally reimbursed by Medicare or Medicaid. Patients eligible for Medicaid could receive both waivered and regular Medicare and Medicaid services while patients who qualified for Medicare only could receive both waivered and regular Medicare services. Since all patients qualified for waivered benefits if eligible for Medicare and/or Medicaid, and had the same services in the same geographic area available to them, the treatment and control groups differed only in the model of case management used. The treatment group received case management from Neighborhood Teams while Centralized Individual case managers provided case management to the control group as well as to the rest of their caseload.

The Centralized Individual case managers were nurses or social workers, and were assisted by case aides. The case aides performed clerical functions, calculated the costs of patient care plans, and contacted service providers to arrange, alter, or discontinue services.

Each of the two Neighborhood Teams consisted of a nurse, social worker, and case aide. Both the nurse and the social worker on the Team functioned as a case manager and delivered a limited amount of direct services as qualified. Inspired by the Kent Community Care Project in England (Davies and Challis, 1980; Davies and Challis, 1986), the Neighborhood Team model was designed to provide a multidisciplinary case management approach which operated as a "true" team in a specific catchment area as well as to allow for more autonomy and independence. Other incentives were provided by reducing the size of the caseload carried by each case manager (from 120-150 skilled nursing and intermediate care level patients to 40-45 skilled nursing level patients) and by routinely visiting patients and informal caregivers at home. It was anticipated that the nurse would incorporate more of a social work perspective and techniques by making home visits with the social worker, and that the social worker would gain more of the nursing perspective. This model would therefore operate more as a team than those in several of the demonstration projects referred to above in which the social worker and nurse would neither have co-responsibility for a case nor make home visits together.

Table 1 presents significant contrasts between the Centralized Individual and Neighborhood Team models. These include home visiting, caseload size, continuity of assessments, familiarity with and counseling of informal caregivers, and autonomy and independence.

Home Visits

Under the Individual Model, many functions, including patient assessment and reassessment, care plan development, and service delivery, were delegated to health care providers (principally certified home health agency and hospital nurses and social workers) rather than performed by employees of the case management organization (i.e., ACCESS). Thus, the case manager depended on completed patient assessment forms and care plans as well as telephone calls from health care providers and clients to manage her clients' care. She rarely visited clients at home. This resulted in Individual Model case managers reacting to changes in clients' conditions and development of problems after they occurred.

On the other hand, Neighborhood Team case managers had first-hand information about client problems gathered during home visits. The Team case manager could visit a client immediately if her condition changed or a problem arose, and did not need to rely solely on information from others. The close contact that the Neighborhood Team case manager maintained with her clients allowed for more timely changes in care plans when a client's needs changed. This was intended to encourage early discharge of clients from hospitals, minimize unnecessary long term nursing home placement, and promote client referrals to rehabilitation and other community-based care programs whenever possible. Home visits by the Team case managers also allowed them to work to prevent client problems or resolve them in their earliest stages. Because the case managers were able to respond quickly to problems, clients frequently called them as soon as a problem occurred. This often allowed the case manager to intervene before the situation reached a crisis.

Caseload Per Case Manager

Having a reasonable caseload per case manager is essential in allowing the case manager sufficient time to perform the tasks necessary to reduce unnecessary formal healthcare service utilization. In the Individual Model, ACCESS case managers have traditionally had quite large caseloads, ranging from 70 to 80 skilled level clients per case manager in addition to an approximately equal number of intermediate and domiciliary care level clients. On the other hand, each Neighborhood Team had a caseload of an average of only 85 patients *per team*, or 40 to 45 per case manager, with no intermediate or domiciliary care level patients. The purpose of lower caseloads was to enable Team case managers to work more intensively with patients and their families, including making home visits as frequently as necessary.

Continuity of Assessments

The issue of continuity between the original assessment of a patient and later reassessments is one that is seldom recognized. In the Individual Model, the first reassessment was usually not conducted by the nurse who completed the original assessment. Later reassessments were often carried out by still other nurses. The nurse assessors would be less likely to modify the amount of formal services if they had not previously assessed the patient. The Individual Model case manager could only question the nurse assessor and have the recommended service plan modified if the degree of patient change was readily apparent from the written reassessment.

In the Neighborhood Team Model, reassessments were almost always done by the nurse who had conducted the initial assessment. As the Team case manager had directly observed the client's condition and how it had changed over time, she was more willing than the Individual Model nurse assessor to reduce the level of formal services as the patient's condition improved. She was also more willing to suggest alternatives, such as substituting day care for eight hours of aide service. The social worker case manager concentrated on informal caregiver assessment while the nurse case manager focused on the patient assessment. By becoming more aware of the other discipline's perspective through working to-

TABLE 1. Contrasts Between Centralized Individual and Neighborhood Team Models

	Centralized Individual Model	Neighborhood Team
(1) Home Visits	Case manager seldom makes visits; depends on others to report problems	Makes visits as often as needed; sees patient/family in home situation firsthand
(2) Caseload	120-150 per case manager	40-45 per case manager
(3) Continuity of Assessments	Reassessments often done by different nurse assessors	Reassessments almost always done by initial Team nurse assessor
(4) Identification and Resolution of Problems Regarding Nurses Aides	Less control as others must report problems	Can identify problems during home visits
(5) Problems of Informal Caregivers	Not as aware of problems or as effective in counseling	More aware of problems and more effective in counseling and teaching
(6) Application for Medicaid	Case manager advises family where to apply and what to do	Case manager sometimes assists client with paperwork and accompanies client to Medicaid office

(7) Supplies and Equipment	If client has questions, answers or refers to vendor	Verifies appropriateness of equipment and its use or administration during visits
(8) Nursing Home Placement	Offers alternatives over the telephone and refers to social workers	Meets personally with clients and families and helps them with their decision
(9) Financial and Legal Problems	If advise is sought, refers to financial counselor or Adult Protective Services	Becomes more aware of problems through visiting; assists clients to ensure problems are resolved
(10) Crisis Situations	Usually not made aware until crisis occurs; intervention more difficult and less effective	Can see crisis developing over time; can intervene more easily, rapidly, and effectively
(11) Geographic Area	Larger area	Smaller area; gets to know local resources better
(12) Autonomy and Independence	Less autonomy and independence	More autonomy and independence
(13) Hospitalization	Transfers case to hospital case manager; unable to advocate for patient	Team visits during hospitalization; supports patient/family; advocates for appropriate discharge plan

gether, each was better able to perform a more comprehensive assessment.

Identification and Resolution of Problems
Regarding Nurses Aides

While both Individual and Team Model case managers were notified by telephone of problems with nurses aides or of difficulties between patients and aides, Team case managers could much more often personally observe aide service during home visits (which were often unannounced). In addition, the greater rapport that Team case managers presumably had with families could lead to a greater likelihood of these issues being raised by families. Because they did not know their case managers as well, patients managed by Individual Model case managers were more likely to fear that services might be discontinued if they raised questions or issues about their care.

In situations where too many hours of aide service were being provided, the Team case managers were better able to change these care plans and reduce the cost of aide service. In other cases less costly services, such as increased use of informal caregivers and social day care, were substituted for aide service. Team case managers were able in other instances to keep care plans at adequate levels despite requests for increased service.

Problems of Informal Caregivers

During home visits the Team case managers could discuss in person with the informal caregivers problems the caregivers and other family members were having including medical, financial, psychological, legal, and other concerns. The Team case manager could become an advocate for an informal caregiver when a care plan was in danger of deterioration because the caregiver was unable to deal with his or her own problems. The informal caregivers were the primary responsibility and concern of the social worker case manager because of her particular expertise.

Application for Medicaid

Both the Individual and Team Model case managers discussed the possibility of applying for Medicaid with their patients/families. Upon request, the Individual Model case managers advised patients and informal caregivers about the Medicaid application process. In contrast, the Team case managers could be much more involved in assisting the client in actually completing the Medicaid application and gathering the necessary documentation because the case manager would visit the patient at home. When it appeared that the client/family might be overwhelmed by the application process, the Team case manager could go with the client to their Medicaid appointment. Because of her expertise, assistance with Medicaid applications would be the primary responsibility of the social worker case manager.

Supplies and Equipment

When the patient or informal caregiver did not understand how to use a piece of equipment and telephoned the Individual Model case manager for information, the case manager could provide directions or refer them to the vendor. When the equipment was inappropriate, the case manager had the vendor deliver the correct supplies and return the incorrect item. In contrast, the Team case manager could visit the client at home to personally verify problems regarding supplies or equipment and/or instruct the patient or caregiver on their proper usage. On the Team, eligibility and use of supplies and equipment were primarily the function of the nurse case manager while payment issues were primarily handled by the social worker. Either might be involved if there was a problem with delivery. The social worker had the responsibility to research payers and mobilize resources.

Nursing Home Admission

Both Individual and Team case managers were aware of Medicaid and private pay clients who were seeking admission to a nursing home. The Individual case managers were more reactive than proactive because they only rarely made home visits. Over the telephone the Individual case managers could offer alternatives to nursing home admission to clients and families. They contacted social workers under contract to ACCESS who then would counsel patients and families and would sometimes fill out nursing home application forms.

The Team case managers were more proactive because they could see the patient's condition with their own eyes. They could meet directly with clients, families, and caretakers to determine whether a client really wanted to be admitted to a nursing home, and could offer alternatives to admission such as day care, respite, or alternative housing. In some cases the case manager acted as a client advocate when a client preferred to remain at home but the family wanted placement. In other cases the Team case managers helped and supported the patient and family during the placement process. The Team would jointly discuss the situation before making a recommendation to the patient and/or family. The social worker case manager would actually assist the patient and/or family with the application.

Financial and Legal Problems

When financial or legal advice was sought by clients or families, in both models the case managers could refer them to a financial counselor. In the Team model, the social worker case managers could directly assist the clients in straightening out problems such as bill-paying or applying for Food Stamps or Supplemental Security Income. Where there were lengthy waits of one year or longer to process requests for conservatorships, money management, and other legal services provided by the Department of Social Services, the Team staff found a local private attorney who was able to process paper work for a conservatorship in about one month.

Crisis Situations

There were two advantages of the Team regarding crisis situations. First, the Team model was more of a preventive approach. The case manager often saw crises in their earlier stages as she made home visits and was more able to prevent their continued development. Second, the Team case manager could be more effective in dealing with crises once they developed. She usually knew the client and family better and could more rapidly intervene. The nature of the crisis situation primarily determined whether the nurse or social worker case manager was involved, although sometimes (i.e., in unexpected crises) it was totally dependent on whomever was making the visit.

In some crisis situations case managers worked closely with a social worker from the Rochester Police Department Family Assistance Team. While the Individual case manager sometimes went to the client's home with the Police Department social worker, the Team case manager always tried to do so.

Geographic Area

While the Individual Model case managers served patients scattered throughout the entire county, the Neighborhood Team provided case management in a limited geographic area. This enabled them to get to know local resources both better and more personally. The Team also could develop a closer identification with the neighborhood and a better ability to work with local organizations such as churches and senior groups.

Autonomy and Independence

The Team had greater control over their operations than the Individual Model case managers. They had more autonomy and independence in managing the care of their patients, which presumably led to greater professional satisfaction on the part of the Team case managers as compared with the Individual case managers.

Hospitalization

The two models differed greatly in their contacts and interactions with patients/families when patients were hospitalized. In the Individual Model, the case was transferred to the hospital case manager for the hospital to which the patient was admitted. (Hospital case managers were ACCESS employees who were stationed in each hospital to facilitate assessments, care planning, and transfer to a nursing home or home care upon discharge.) The hospital case manager was of course not as familiar with a patient and his or her family as the case manager responsible for the patient when the patient was living at home.

In the Team model, ACCESS's responsibility for the case remained with the Team when the patient was in the hospital. Except in situations where the patient was in the hospital for only a brief stay for a "routine" diagnostic procedure or treatment (e.g., chemotherapy) or for observation (e.g., after falling), one or both members of the Team would visit the patient in the hospital. A Team member would usually meet with family members at the hospital or at home. The Team would assist the hospital discharge planner to expedite discharge. By maintaining continuity in their relationship with the family, the Team was more likely to be able to facilitate earlier discharge.

The Team also believed that patients age 90 and over were more likely to be restrained and sedated than younger patients, and less likely to be considered candidates for rehabilitation. Therefore, the Team more aggressively intervened on behalf of these patients. In many cases the Team would request that the patient be transferred to the special demonstration rehabilitation unit for elderly patients at one of the local hospitals.

Evaluation of Effectiveness

The Neighborhood Team model (273 cases) was more cost-effective than the Individual model (203 cases) over the two-year period of the study. Total estimated health care expenditures were 14% less per patient per day for Team patients. Both hospital and home care use and costs were lower (26% and 24%, respectively) while nursing home use/costs were greater (48%). The latter was due, at least in part, to substitution of nursing home days for hospital days. Mortality was very high, and about the same for both groups during the first year after entry into the study (30%), but lower for the Team during the second year (11% as compared with 16%), using a life table-survivorship analysis. Patient and caregiver satisfaction and patient morale did not differ significantly (Eggert, Zimmer, Hall, and Friedman, 1989). The Team also appeared to have a delaying effect on patients becoming Medicaid eligible. Of those entering the study not Medicaid eligible, 43% fewer Team cases went on Medicaid during the study (adjusted for length of time in the study).

DEMENTIA PATIENTS AND CASE MANAGEMENT INTERVENTIONS IN THE ACCESS STUDY

A number of secondary analyses of the ACCESS case management study data were conducted to determine how the effects of the Team and Individual case management models differed between various diagnostic and demographic subgroups. Among all subgroups examined, patients having dementia were found to have experienced the greatest reductions in health care utilization and costs under Team case management. A retrospective chart review was carried out on this group to determine what specific activities and interventions of case management differed between the two models. The dementia patients were analyzed since it would be likely that the difference would be the most obvious in the group with the greatest cost reductions.

Among the cases with dementia, total estimated health care expenditures for the 46 Team patients were 41% lower than for the 48 patients managed by the Centralized Individual Model. As with the entire group, hospital and home care utilization and expenditures were substantially lower for Team patients, but even more so, at 69% less for hospital care and 47% less for home care. Nursing home use/costs was about the same for both Team and Control dementia patients. Ambulatory care utilization was much higher (275%) for Team cases, but accounted for only a small proportion of total costs. Greater day care use with the associated chairmobile rides accounted for most of the latter. No differences were found between the two models regarding mortality, functional and care need status, and caregiver satisfaction (Zimmer, Eggert, and Chiverton, 1989).

Why was the Neighborhood Team approach more cost-effective? From the chart review of the dementia cases, it appears that several factors were responsible. First, as was intended by the intervention, Team case managers made considerably more visits to the patients, principally at home (80% of all visits), but also to other locations. Team case managers provided 18 times more visits per patient per year (5.5) than case managers in the Centralized Individual model (0.3). Second, Team case managers made 31% more referrals to other providers or services. Higher proportions of Team patients than control patients were referred for medical evaluation (46% as compared to 27%), overnight respite care (33% versus 19%), day care (17% as compared to 2%), and financial planning (35% versus 19%). Third, higher proportions of Team patients received counseling from case managers for family support (61% as compared to 6%) and service availability and access (78% versus 42%) (Zimmer, Eggert, and Chiverton, 1989).

HOME HEALTH CARE TEAM STUDY

The third model of "Intensive Case Management" (see Figure 1) discussed in this paper is the Home Health Care Team (HHCT) developed as an outreach program of the University of Rochester Medical Center's Ambulatory Care Unit in 1977. (The HHCT is now based at St. John's Home.) Since its establishment, the HHCT has consisted of a physician specializing in geriatric medicine, a geriatric nurse practitioner, and a medical social worker. The HHCT was organized to provide primary care at home to homebound chronically and terminally ill elderly patients, and has been on call 24 hours per day, seven days per week.

A randomized controlled evaluation was funded by the National Center for Health Services Research from 1978 to 1981 (Zimmer, Groth-Juncker, and McCusker, 1985). In order to be eligible for care by the HHCT, patients had to be homebound, desire to continue to live at home, have significant illness (not primarily psychiatric) requiring medical care, have had a physician who did not wish to make home visits, and have an informal caregiver (family member or friend) who could significantly participate in caring for them at home. About one-fifth of HHCT patients had a prognosis of terminal status (Zimmer, Groth-Juncker, and McCusker, 1985). Patients were randomized into the Treatment Group (81 cases), which received care from the HHCT or the Control Group (75 cases), which received care as normally provided in the community. "In most cases, the difference between study group care and control group care revolved around the availability of the geriatric physician and the nurse practitioner for home-based medical visits" (Groth-Juncker, 1988).

The Home Health Care Team operated differently from the Neighborhood Team in a number of ways. First, unlike the Neighborhood Team, members of the HHCT rarely made joint visits. Second, the HHCT social worker almost always made the initial visit. The initial visit of the Neighborhood Team was usually a joint one. Third, in the HHCT the geriatric nurse practitioner was always the supervisor of the community health nurse (CHN) who was not a member of the HHCT and delivered the majority of routine nursing services. In the Neighborhood Team neither of the case managers was the supervisor of the CHN. Fourth, in the HHCT the nurse supervised the home health or personal care aide. In the Neighborhood Team the aide was supervised by the CHN, not the Team case managers. Fifth, while both members of the Neighborhood Team assisted and supported the patient and family during the nursing home placement process, in the HHCT the social worker did most of this. Finally, the social worker in both the Neighborhood Team and HHCT functioned very similarly regarding problems of informal caregivers, applications for Medicaid, supplies and equipment, and financial and legal problems.

Hospital utilization, adjusted for days at risk, was 38% lower for HHCT patients (2.04 days per patient per month) than for control group patients (3.29 days) during the six months of the study. Nursing home use was 58% lower for HHCT patients (0.55 days per person per month as compared with 1.32 days for the controls). Physician office visits and clinic visits were both lower (70% and 79%, respectively) but emergency room visits were five times as great (.26 per patient per month for HHCT patients as compared with .05 for the controls). As would be expected, in-home health services utilization was greater for persons receiving care from the HHCT. This was especially so for physician home visits (almost eight times greater for Home Health Care Team patients), social worker visits (four times greater), LPN hours (6.6 times as many), and home laboratory technician visits (nine times greater). Total health care expenditures were estimated to be 8.6% lower for patients cared for by the HHCT, but this difference was not statistically significant (Zimmer, Groth-Juncker, and McCusker, 1985).

HOME HEALTH CARE TEAM AND TERMINAL CARE

The lower health care expenditures estimated for persons managed by the HHCT were almost entirely due to lower costs among the patients who died. These were compared for those who had died (21 HHCT patients and 16 controls) and those who were alive at three months after study entry (60 HHCT patients and 59 controls). While the average per diem costs of HHCT patients who were alive were only 2% lower than those of the controls, those of HHCT patients who had died were 26% lower than those of deceased control group members (Zimmer, Groth-Juncker, and McCusker, 1984).

Utilization data were examined for the last two weeks of life of 33 patients who died and were in the study for at least that amount of time. The 21 patients cared for by the HHCT spent about half as many days in the hospital during the terminal two weeks (3.1 days) as compared to the 12 control group members (6.1 days). Only 29% of HHCT were in the hospital during the last two weeks in comparison with 58% of the control group. HHCT patients had greater average utilization for physician home visits (0.8 versus 0.1), nurse home visits (1.7 as compared to 1.1), RN/LPN hours (51.2 versus 42.0), and aide/homemaker visits (21.1 versus 11.5). Neither group entered a nursing home during the terminal period. Average estimated total costs during the last two weeks of life were almost one-third (31%) lower for HHCT patients (Zimmer, Groth-Juncker, and McCusker, 1984).

Among patients dying within six months of study entry, almost twice as great a proportion of Home Health Care Team patients died at home (71%) as did control group patients (41%). Interviews with caregivers after the patients' death found significantly greater satisfaction with HHCT care, especially for availability of care, pain control, and general satisfaction with care provided (Zimmer, Groth-Juncker, and McCusker, 1984).

COMPARISON OF THE THREE MODELS

Studies of mental health case management often do not clearly define the components of different models of case management. "Without such information, effectiveness comparisons across programs are meaningless because it is not clear what is being compared" (Baker and Intagliata, 1989). This is also true in long term care. They also point out that "standardized operational definitions" of case management are needed to allow comparisons. Again, this is true for long term care case management. Accordingly, we have modified Ross's (1980) framework and included our three intensive case management models as well as his minimal and comprehensive models (see Table 2).

In examining Table 2 one can see that the Home Health Care Team is the most intensive of the three models reviewed in this article, followed by the Neighborhood Team and then the Centralized Individual Model. The three models differ principally in the functions of client assessment and reassessment, direct service, and crisis intervention.

- *Client Assessment and Reassessment*: The Home Health Care Team performs all three types of client assessment (medical, nursing, and social work) while the Neighborhood Team delegates one (medical) and performs two (nursing and social work). In the Centralized Individual Model all three are delegated. While reassessments are performed by one or more members of the HHCT and the Neighborhood Team, in the Centralized Individual Model they are delegated to other providers, principally community health nurses.
- *Direct Services*: The HHCT provides medical, social work, and some nursing service, while the Neighborhood Team delegates medical care and provides social work and some nursing. The Centralized Individual Model delegates all three direct services.
- *Crisis Intervention*: The HHCT can provide the most crisis intervention in the home, the Neighborhood Team some, and the Centralized Individual Model the least.

TABLE 2. Case Management Models

Functions[a]	Comprehensive Model[a]	Home Health Care Team
Outreach	Yes	No
Client assessment	Yes	
° Medical		Yes
° Nursing		Yes
° Social work		Yes
Care planning	Yes	Yes
Referral to service providers	Yes	Yes
Advocacy for client	Yes	Yes
Direct service	Yes	
° Medical		Yes
° Nursing		Shared
° Social work		Yes
Developing natural support systems	Yes	Yes
Reassessment	Yes	Yes
Advocacy for resource development	Yes	No
Monitoring quality	Yes	Proactive
Public education	Yes	No
Crisis intervention	Yes	More

[a]Source: Modified from Ross (1980)

Neighborhood Team Model	Centralized Individual Model	Minimal Model
No	No	Yes
		Yes
Delegated	Delegated	
Yes	Delegated	
Yes	Delegated	
Yes	Delegated	Yes
Yes	Yes	Yes
Yes	Yes	No
		No
Delegated	No	
Shared	No	
Yes	No	
Yes	Limited	No
Yes	Delegated	No
No	No	No
Proactive	Reactive	No
Yes	No	No
Intermediate	Less	No

LESSONS LEARNED

Our experience in developing, managing, and evaluating case management models as well as our review of the literature have taught us a number of lessons. First, not everyone needs case management. It has become such a popular concept that the care system seems to be on a course to provide it to every person who requires some health or social services. This will prove to be highly unnecessary as well as very cost-ineffective. Second, different models of case management are more effective and efficient than other models for different types of patients with different prognoses. Identification of the benefits and disadvantages of specific models for specific types of patients has begun.

As with the use of home and community-based care to substitute for nursing home or hospital care (Eggert and Friedman, 1988), targeting is the key to determining which types of patients might benefit from various types of case management. The Neighborhood Team model begins to do this for dementia patients as does the HHCT model for terminal care patients. As part of the targeting process, the following levels of case management intensity can be suggested:

- Provide only information and referral
- Train patients and/or informal caregivers to perform various case management tasks
- Provide case management for limited periods of time and/or of limited intensity
- Provide ongoing intensive case management

The following elaborates on each of these levels. First, some patients/informal caregivers require only information and referral. Their needs and capabilities are such that only a minimal "intervention" of this type is necessary. Most elderly people, including some who are quite chronically ill, presumably "fit" in this category.

Second, other patients/informal caregivers can be trained to perform various case management functions (Seltzer, Ivry, and Litchfield, 1987). Many individuals, including those who are chronically ill, can perform many of these tasks. The closeness and degree of monitoring by the case manager of the performance of each task depends on the competence and attentiveness of the informal caregiver.

Third, case management can be time-limited. It can be provided for shorter or longer periods of time depending upon the severity of illness, its stability, the patient's prognosis, and the ability of the patient/primary informal caregiver to learn case management tasks. For example, patients in the ACCESS:Medicare demonstration program received active case management for an average of 56 days each time they received ACCESS:Medicare benefits. For the remainder of the time many who were in the demonstration were contacted by telephone only once every six months to check on their health status.

Fourth, some individuals will require ongoing intensive case management. For them, this might be performed by an individual, a two-person team, or a large multidisciplinary team. Depending on the diagnoses, condition, prognosis, and ability of the patient and informal caregiver, home visits can be scheduled more or less frequently, different types of assessments can be performed, various types of professionals or paraprofessionals can contact the patient/ informal caregiver in person, by telephone, or by mail, and several types of interventions (e.g., counseling) can be performed by those carrying out the various case management tasks.

Decisions as to which level of case management intensity is indicated require both an initial triage system and an effective ongoing monitoring system to detect the need for changes in that level of case management. Only then can properly targeted case management and efficient service delivery be accomplished.

REFERENCES

Baker, F., and J. Intagliata. (In press). Case management of the seriously mentally ill. In R.P. Liberman (Ed.), *Rehabilitation of the seriously mentally ill*. New York: Plenum.

Barker, W., T. Williams, J. Zimmer, C. Van Buren, S. Vincent, and S. Pickrel. (1985). Geriatric consultation teams in acute hospitals: Impact on back-up of elderly patients. *Journal of the American Geriatrics Society*, 33, 422-428.

Davies, B., and D. Challis. (1988). Experimenting with new roles in domiciliary service: The Kent Community Care Project. *The Gerontologist*, 20, 288-299.

Davies, B., and D. Challis. (1986). *Matching resource to needs in community* care: An evaluated demonstration of a long-term care model. Hants, England: Gower Publishing Company Limited.

Eggert, G., J. Bowlyow, and C. Nichols. (1980). Gaining control of the long term care system: First returns from the ACCESS experiment. *The Gerontologist*, 20, 356-363.

Eggert, G., and B. Friedman. (1988). The need for special interventions for multiple hospital admission patients. *Health Care Financing Review*, Annual Supplement, 57-67.

Eggert, G., J. Zimmer, W.J. Hall, and B. Friedman. (Submitted for publication). Case management: A randomized controlled study comparing a neighborhood team and a centralized individual model.

Groth-Juncker, A. (1988). Ten essentials for a successful home health-care team. *HMO Practice* 2, 47-52.

Kemper, P., R. Applebaum, and M. Harrigan. (1987). Community care demonstrations: What have we learned? *Health Care Financing Review*, 8, 87-100.

Mailick Seltzer, M., J. Ivry, and L. Litchfield. (1987). Family members as case managers: Partnership between the formal and informal support networks. *The Gerontologist*, 27, 722-728.

Ross, H. (1980). *Proceedings of the conference on the evaluation of case management programs, March 5-6, 1979*. Los Angeles: Volunteers for Service to Older Persons.

University of Rochester. (1968). *Health Care of Aged Study: A Study of the Physical and Mental Health Care Needs of Older People in Monroe County, New York*. Rochester, N.Y.: Department of Preventive Medicine, School of Medicine and Dentistry, University of Rochester.

Weissert, W., C. Matthews Cready, and J. Pawelak. (1988). The past and future of home- and community-based long-term care. *The Milbank Quarterly*, 66, 309-388.

Wenkert, W., and M. Terris. (1960). Methods and findings in a local chronic illness study. *American Journal of Public Health*, 50, 1288-1297.

Wenkert, W., J. Hill, and R. Berg. (1979). Concepts and methodology in planning patient care services. *Medical Care*, 7, 327-331.

Williams, M., T. Williams, J. Zimmer, W. Hall, and C. Podgorski. (1987). How does the team approach to outpatient geriatric evaluation compare with traditional care: A report of a randomized controlled trial. *Journal of the American Geriatrics Society*, 35, 1071-1078.

Williams, T., J. Hill, M. Fairbank, and K. Knox. (1973). Appropriate placement of the chronically ill and aged: A successful approach by evaluation. *JAMA*, 226, 1332-1335.

Zimmer, J. (1987). Institutional and community approaches in planning services for the elderly. Presented at U.S.-Israel Cooperation in Health — Fourth Binational Symposium: The Challenge of Aging Societies. Bethesda, MD, National Institutes of Health, Nov. 15-17. Summary: (1988). *Public Health Reports*, 103, 515-547.

Zimmer, J., G. Eggert, and P. Chiverton. (Submitted for publication). Individual vs team case management in optimizing community care for chronically ill patients with dementia.

Zimmer, J., A. Groth-Juncker, and J. McCusker. (1984). Effects of a physician-led home care team on terminal care. *Journal of the American Geriatrics Society*, 32, 288-292.

Zimmer, J., A. Groth-Juncker, and J. McCusker. (1985). A randomized controlled study of a home health care team. *American Journal of Public Health*, 75, 134-141.

Community-Based Long Term Care: The Experience of the Living at Home Programs

Susan L. Hughes
Marylou Guihan

SUMMARY. Through the Living at Home Program (LAHP) 20 communities across the United States have developed cooperative networks involving multiple health and social services providers. The LAHP networks have sought to increase access to care, reduce duplication of services, and identify and fill service gaps. The LAHP national evaluation is examining the inter-organizational linkages that have been implemented by the networks and the characteristics of 1500 clients enrolled for care.

Preliminary findings at the midpoint of the evaluation indicate that the networks have moved from a reliance on informal communication and coordination mechanisms at baseline to the use of more formal structural mechanisms over time. Despite the lack of formal targeting criteria, the networks have enrolled a quite frail elderly population. Future analyses will examine variability across the networks in client targeting and service utilization, in order to shed light on the need for utilization review of community based long term care.

Even under conditions of severe dependency and terminal illness, 70% of older Americans prefer to receive long term care at home (Louis Harris and Associates, 1982). The cost-effectiveness of community-based long term care has been examined exhaustively

---

Correspondence may be addressed to the first author (Susan L. Hughes) at: CHSPR, Northwestern University, 629 Noyes Street, Evanston, IL 60208.

This publication was supported by a grant from The Commonwealth Fund (grant # 10448). In all cases, the statements made and the views expressed are those of the authors and do not reflect those of The Commonwealth Fund.

103

over the last 20 years, resulting in largely equivocal findings (Kemper et al., 1987, Weissert 1985a, Hughes, 1985). Although no clear evidence exists regarding cost savings, these studies have yielded important information about the size and characteristics of the community-based long term care population (Weissert, 1985b). In short, the size of the community-based long term care population does not appear to be overwhelming and the repeated documentation of its unmet needs for care argue that some method (whether public, private or some combination of the two) can and should be developed to finance a system of care.

At present, several alternative financing methods have been proposed, including a proposal by the Commonwealth Commission on the Elderly Living Alone. These proposals are being reviewed by Congressional staff and by the Pepper Commission. A consensus seems to have emerged that a need for care exists, and that the dimensions of equitable methods of financing this care can be identified. What is less clear, is the shape that the delivery system for such care would assume. Data from the community care demonstrations consistently show that frail elderly in the community have a large variety of unmet needs for a combination of health and social services that are currently provided by two separate and parallel service systems (Hughes, 1986). Many have argued that some case or care management function should be developed to increase access to and coordinate services across our multiple and complex sets of care providers. Binstock (1987) has proposed a uniform delivery system of Aging Resource Centers for Help (ARCHs) that would use the existing national network of Area Agencies on Aging to assess clients and coordinate their care. While this strategy has the advantage of designating a single responsible case management source, it might also be somewhat premature as a society to lock ourselves into a uniform system of public case managers, especially since competent voluntary providers in many communities have been providing this function for many years. The question then appears to be, can we capitalize upon the diversity and expertise that is inherent in our existing delivery system or should we impose an oversight system upon it in order to ensure equitable access to care and the efficient allocation of resources.

The experience of the Living at Home Program (LAHP), a national demonstration that is currently being conducted in twenty communities across the United States (shown in Appendix 1), may shed some light on some of these important questions. LAHP is attempting to demonstrate that cooperative networks of health and social services providers can reduce duplication of and increase access to existing services. LAHP was initiated by the Commonwealth Fund and the Pew Charitable Trusts and has since grown to encompass a 7.5 million dollar demonstration that is co-sponsored by a uniquely broad-based coalition of 33 additional charitable foundations.

The LAHP Program Office is headed by Morton Bogdonoff, M.D. at the New York Hospital-Cornell Medical Center. The 18 member National Advisory Committee is chaired by Robert N. Butler, M.D. of Mount Sinai Medical Center in New York. The three-year LAHP demonstration began in 1987 at 20 different sites across the United States which had a minimum population of 200,000 persons (Table 1).

LAHP attempted to capitalize upon the synergism that results when agencies cooperate rather than compete. The basic theory behind LAHP was that community-based medical and social services are scarce and the number of elderly persons requiring them is growing. To avoid duplication of scarce services and manpower, at each site a Lead Agency was funded to implement a voluntary network of Affiliate Agencies whose joint task was to streamline access to care for the elderly, reduce duplication of services, identify consistent service gaps and devise innovative ways of filling them.

The LAHP demonstration sites were purposely selected to test a variety of new approaches to the organization and management of community-based care. Researchers at Northwestern University's Center for Health Services and Policy Research have been conducting the national evaluation. They have been collaborating with another research team headed by William Weissert, Ph.D. at the University of Michigan, which has provided technical assistance to the demonstration sites in the areas of prospective budgeting and service supply and demand estimation.

To date, the Northwestern group has identified three different models of care that are subsumed by the LAHP umbrella (Table 1). Approximately six "outreach/access" sites attempted to reach

TABLE 1

CITY	CATCHMENT AREA	INTERVENTION TYPE	TYPE OF AGENCY
Boston (1)	Neighborhood	Outreach/CM	Hospital
Boston (2)	Neighborhood	Outreach/CM	Community Health Center
Buffalo	County	CM	Case Management Agency
Charlotte	City	Respite/Meals	Hospital
Chicago	City	Respite	Social Services
Cincinnati	County	Information System	A.A.A.
Denver	County	CM	Case Management Agency
Durham	Neighborhood	Volunteer/CM	Social Services
Miami	County	Short Term CM	Residential Care
Milwaukee	City	Volunteer/CM	Case Management Agency
Nashville	City	CM	Social Services

New York (1)	Neighborhood	Outreach/CM	Hospital
New York (2)	Neighborhood	Volunteer/CM	Hospital
New York (3)	Neighborhood	Outreach/CM	Social Services
Oklahoma City	County	CM	A.A.A.
Pasadena	City	Outreach	Hospital
Pittsburgh	City	CM	Hospital
St. Paul	Neighborhood	Volunteer/CM	Home Care Agency
San Francisco	City	Outreach /CM	Residential Care
Tucson	County	CM	A.A.A.

CM= Case Management

groups that previously may have lacked access to organized community-based care. Two of these sites, South Cove Community Health Center in Boston and St. Vincent's Chelsea Village Program in New York, targeted services to frail inner-city elderly Chinese. The East Harlem Council for Human Services targeted services to elderly Hispanics. San Francisco's Northern California Presbyterian Homes Services for Seniors placed outreach resident advocates in Tenderloin area single room occupancy hotels and three other senior housing sites (public and private). Pasadena's Senior Care Network provided outreach service to resistant clients and Boston's University Hospital Elders Living at Home Program served elderly at risk of becoming homeless.

Other programs attempted to augment scarce professional expertise by joining forces with paraprofessionals, volunteer outreach workers and/or family caregivers. St. Paul's Ramsey County Public Health Nursing Service worked with two neighborhood community councils to provide community volunteers for outreach and information and referral, with more complex case management being provided by back-up Public Health block nurses. Durham's Coordinating Council for Senior Citizens and Pittsburgh's Montefiore Hospital used trained paraprofessional "Neighborhood Advisors" and Milwaukee's Community Care Organization used inter-faith caregivers from a consortium of religious congregations to provide similar kinds of "front and hot line" assistance. In contrast, Chicago's Council for the Jewish Elderly and Charlotte's Presbyterian Hospital Senior Care Network concentrated on the development of new in-home and in-patient respite services.

Other sites attempted to reduce duplication of services by developing a common assessment tool for use by all agencies in the network and/or by developing and sharing an automated database on volunteers and other community services. Finally, the Short Term Emergency Services program sponsored by Miami Jewish Home and Hospital for the Aged, tested the innovative notion of short term emergency case management with an average per client expenditure cap of $350. The intent at this site was to determine whether a limited investment during a crisis could link clients to appropriate services, thereby forestalling the need for a more prolonged and expensive alternative care plan.

EVALUATION DESIGN

The design that is being used to evaluate LAHP sought to capitalize upon the diversity inherent in the demonstration sites. The first phase of the design used a repeat organizational change survey to examine the availability of services and the ways in which Lead Agencies and their Affiliates collaborated before, at the mid-point and at the end of the demonstration.

The number of agencies in each LAHP network at baseline ranged from a low of two to a high of 80. The organizational change survey was mailed to all Lead Agencies and to all Affiliates if the network contained 10 or fewer Affiliates. If the network contained more than 10 Affiliates, the Lead Agencies were asked to identify the set of 10 Affiliates with whom they interacted most frequently. This resulted in a sampling frame of 20 Lead Agencies and 160 Affiliate Agencies for a total nationwide sample of 180 health and social service providers.

The baseline organizational change survey asked respondents to describe conditions that prevailed in their communities prior to the inception of LAHP. The mid-point (Time 2) survey examined changes that occurred over approximately one and a half years of the demonstration. Response rates to the surveys were very high at 100% for Time 1 and 98% for Time 2.

During Year Three, repeat administration of the organizational change survey will ascertain which types of coordination mechanisms are more successful in identifying and filling service gaps. These data will also yield information about service gaps that persist, for which more global state or national legislation or funding may be required.

The second "process" phase of the evaluation has sought to define the Living at Home client and to examine variability in community care service utilization. For this purpose, all sites were requested to complete a uniform functional assessment on 75 clients who were consecutively accepted for care during Year Two of the demonstration. This "snapshot" of clients taken at a time when referral sources and service operations were in a steady state, was expected to provide valuable information about the range of characteristics that is possible among community care users. During the second year, all sites were also requested to track 12 months of service use by the 75 clients for whom uniform assessment were obtained. These data should enable comparisons of service use across sites, controlling for client risk factors or "case mix." This database will ultimately provide uniform client assessment data on 1,350 community care clients across the United States, together with 12 months of detailed service utilization. Since data collection is still ongoing, this article describes preliminary findings from an examination of the baseline-midpoint organizational change data and preliminary findings from the assessment database.

PRELIMINARY FINDINGS

Characteristics of LAHP Sites

Time 1 organizational change surveys were completed by all 20 Leads and 160 of the Affiliate Agencies in the LAHP networks. The majority (77%) of those who completed surveys were administrators. As Table 1 demonstrates, health and social service providers were evenly represented among the Lead Agencies. The majority of the agencies making up the Affiliate Agencies classified themselves as private social service agencies (35%), followed by public social service agencies (11%), hospitals (11%), other health related agencies (19%) and Areawide Aging Agencies (13%). Thirty two percent classified themselves as "other," which included agencies providing housing and transportation, academic institutions, and for-profit businesses.

For the purpose of governance, 90% of the 20 LAHP sites had set up an Advisory Board or Committee. The Advisory Boards had an average of 15 members, met about 9 times per year and were primarily made up of Affiliate Agencies (64% of Advisory Board members were Affiliates).

The size of geographic catchment areas served by the 20 LAHP sites varied substantially with 20% serving a defined neighborhood, 30% less than city-wide, 25% city-wide and 25% county-wide in scope.

At baseline, the size of the Lead Agency staff varied considerably. The average number of professional staff was 86 FTEs, with a range from 5 to more than 1000. The average number of paraprofessional staff was 155, while the average number of clerical staff was 68 FTEs. However, eighty-five percent of the Lead Agencies had fewer than 80 full-time workers indicating that the mean FTE figures were greatly inflated by the inclusion of Lead Agencies which are hospitals.

Baseline-Midpoint Organization Change. Table 2 examines increases between baseline and the midpoint of the demonstration in percent of services by type that were provided within the Living at Home networks. It indicates across the board expansion in the types and comprehensiveness of community based services that were provided within the networks across the majority of sites. The table also demonstrates a high degree of agreement between Lead and Affiliates agencies regarding those services that increased within the networks. Community-based services (particularly in-home and general support services, which include case management and outreach) increased substantially. The only types of services that did *not* increase were institution-based services, like residential care and nursing home care. This pattern makes sense if one considers that the purpose of the demonstration was to increase services that elderly need to remain in their homes.

Further analysis of specific services (not shown) demonstrated that the service that increased the most was outreach, from 40% at baseline to 85% at the midpoint of the demonstration. It is also worth noting that 65% of the networks provided case management and advocacy at baseline. By the midpoint of the demonstration, as intended, these services were almost universally available (95%) within each Living at Home network.

Table 3 groups different relationships between the Leads and the Affiliates into five major categories and examines change over time. As this table demonstrates, substantial increases occurred over the first year of the demonstration in information sharing and coordination/structure. This is a logical development, given the fact that these types of relationships are somewhat easier to develop than shared budgeting and staff. It is interesting to note, however, that a consistent increase is seen across all five types of relationships that were measured and that in three out of the five instances the Leads

TABLE 2. Services Provided Within the LAHP Network

	Leads		Affiliates	
	Time 1 %	Time 2 %	Time 1 %	Time 2 %
In-home Services	64	80	58	68
General Support (including Case Management & Outreach)	60	80	64	78
Medical Services	53	69	48	57
Medical Facilities	42	55	41	49
Physical Environment (housing repairs, etc.)	35	53	40	28
Financial Services	28	54	40	46
Residential Care	30	36	26	34
Nursing Home Care	30	35	29	35

TABLE 3. Types of Relationships Developed Between Leads and Affiliates

		Leads		Affiliates	
		Time 1 %	Time 2 %	Time 1 %	Time 2 %
1)	Budgeting and Staffing	31	36	14	15
2)	Information Sharing	28	48	22	36
3)	Joint Program Development	40	55	22	22
4)	Coordination/Structure	51	71	40	51
5)	Quality Assurance	18	38	13	18

% for Affiliates reflects the overall response of Affiliates, some of whom may not be as closely linked to the Lead as others.

and Affiliates agree about the types of joint activities that have increased.

What types of coordination mechanisms were used to nurture these relationships? Table 4 indicates that at baseline the main type of coordination mechanism used was an informal one, e.g., direct contact between people or ad hoc group meetings. These activities were still being relied upon heavily at the mid-point of the demonstration. However, the use of formal mechanisms increased substantially. Specifically, the use of written plans and schedules, common assessment forms, rules, policies and procedures, even computerized information systems which are very difficult to develop on a system wide basis, all showed substantial increases with 100% of the Lead Agencies at mid-point reporting the use of common assessment forms within the network.

How do the agencies in the network communicate with one another? Table 5 examines this issue and demonstrates again that at baseline, informal types of communication mechanisms (e.g., telephone discussions and face-to-face meetings) were more frequently used. By the mid-point of the demonstration, a perceptible shift had occurred to the use of more formal types of mechanisms like group problem solving efforts, written reports and regularly scheduled staff meetings.

Data that were presented earlier in Table 2 indicated that substantial increases occurred in the number of community-based services that were provided within the LAHP networks across the sites. Despite this increase in services, Table 6 indicates that barriers to client service use still existed at the mid-point of the demonstration. Ignorance regarding service availability was still ranked a number one problem. The Lead Agencies and the Affiliates also seem to have become more aware of the lack of affordable services over time and to be more cognizant of problems associated with ineligibility for benefits, client self-neglect and unwillingness to pay.

Other data examined indicate that ignorance regarding service availability persisted despite a fair amount of promotional activity. As expected, few of the Lead Agencies used paid TV or radio advertising as promotional mechanisms. However, free advertising was perceived to be as or more effective than paid advertising and a great deal of outreach activity appears to have occurred across the

TABLE 4. Coordination Mechanisms Used

	Leads		Affiliates	
	Time 1 %	Time 2 %	Time 1 %	Time 2 %
Informal				
1. Direct Contact between People	85	100	70	86
2. Ad Hoc Group Meetings	70	70	49	45
3. Board and/or Advisory Board	60	55	46	62
Formal				
1. Written Plans and Schedules	45	80	24	42
2. Common Assessment Forms	45	100	29	70
3. Rules, Policies and Procedures	45	60	22	42
4. Computerized Info. System	25	45	13	29

115

TABLE 5. Communication Mechanisms Used

	Leads		Affiliates	
	Time 1 %	Time 2 %	Time 1 %	Time 2 %
Telephone Discussions	95	100	78	91
Face to Face	95	100	74	92
Group Problem Solving	80	95	51	60
Written Reports	65	75	54	77
Regularly Scheduled Staff Meetings	35	55	19	43

TABLE 6. Client Barriers to Service Use
(Rated as "Frequent" or "Very Frequent")

	Leads		Affiliates	
	Time 1 %	Time 2 %	Time 1 %	Time 2 %
Ignorance Regarding Service	85	85	66	72
Affordability	75	85	51	62
Erroneous Perceptions	70	50	53	51
Waiting Lists	60	55	53	57
Ineligibility	40	55	34	40
Self-Neglect	40	55	33	40
Unwilling to Pay	35	50	33	37
Fear of Stigma	20	50	30	33

demonstration sites with respect to many different types of promotional activities.

Finally, Table 7 examines strategies for continued funding of Living at Home activities after grant funding ceased and indicates a fair amount of activity in this area. The table examines strategies that the sites considered or adopted and the relative effectiveness of those strategies that had been adopted. It indicates that many of the sites have tried sliding scale fees, the development of a private pay market and ties with United Way, as well as the possibility of private foundation support. Not surprisingly, however, those strategies that had been adopted and found most effective were accessing general revenues, obtaining a Medicaid 2176 Waiver contract and obtaining contracts with employers. Although only a small number of sites successfully tapped these funding sources, it appears that these survivability routes should receive high priority from the other sites, perhaps followed by the development of access to Title XX, Title III and county funds. United Way was also perceived as being quite effective by those sites that managed to obtain funding from that source. The Time 3 Organizational Change survey re-examined this issue in September of 1989. It is encouraging to note that by the mid-point of the demonstration, the mean number of strategies adopted was 2.1 across the sites with as many as six strategies already adopted at the Buffalo site. This indicates that the sites were taking survivability seriously and were concentrating their efforts in this area at that point.

To summarize, the comparison of Time 1 and Time 2 organizational change data indicates good correspondence between Leads' and Affiliates' views of the way that the networks function and of their effectiveness. As predicted, system interactions were becoming more formal over time, a necessary development if these networks are to be sustained once Living at Home funding ceases. Also encouraging is the fact that an interpretable pattern has emerged regarding increased types and levels of in-home community-based services that are being provided within the networks, a major goal of the demonstration.

Client Characteristics. Table 8 examines the baseline demographics of Living at Home clients across the 14 sites that had completed functional assessments on more than 50 clients prior to

TABLE 7. Funding Strategies for Post Grant Survival

	Considered (N)	Adopted (N)	Effectiveness (Mean)
Sliding Scale Fees	13	8	3.5
Private Pay Market	12	3	3.7
United Way	12	5	4.4
Private Foundations	12	4	3.5
County Contract	10	5	4.4
General Revenue	9	3	5.0
A.O.A. Title III	7	4	2.5
Medicaid 2176 Waiver	4	2	5.0
Title XX	4	4	4.0
Other State Contract	3	1	2.0
Contracts with Employers	2	2	5.0

Range: 0-6 Adopted   Mean: 2.1 Adopted

TABLE 8. Baseline Demographics: LAHP Clients (N=959)

	Mean or %			
	SOA[a]	LAHP	Channeling[b]	NH[c]
Mean Age	73	78, s.d.=8	80	83
84 Years & Older	7	28	28*	46
Female	59	71	71	75
Married	55	28	32	13
White	90	74	73	93
Living Alone	32	58	37	n/a
Median Household Income				
Per Month	n/a	$535	$649	
Per Year	n/a	$6420	$7788	
Education < 12 Years	49	57	n/a	

* 85+

a. 1984 Supplement on Aging, National Health Interview Survey, National Center for Health Statistics.
b. Applebaum, R. 1988 The Evaluation of the National Long Term Care Demonstration, Recruitment and Characteristics of Channeling Clients. *Health Services Research* 23(1): 51-66.
c. National Nursing Home Survey, National Center for Health Statistics.

4/1/89. This table compares Living at Home clients in the aggregate to other national databases on the elderly. The column that is headed SOA presents data on the Supplement on Aging that was conducted by the National Center for Health Statistics as a supplement to the National Health Interview Survey in 1984. The SOA collected data from a probability sample that represents the total community dwelling elderly population in the United States, regardless of disability status. In contrast, the Channeling column represents the sample of individuals who received care during the National Long Term Care or Channeling Demonstration which used very strict IADL and ADL screening mechanisms to target services to the frail elderly. We expected that the Living at Home clients would fall somewhere between these two populations; i.e., that they would be more impaired than the general U.S. elderly population but less impaired than the Channeling clients because the Living at Home demonstration neither utilized any screening mechanisms consistently across the sites to target impaired clients nor imposed explicit, uniform criteria for acceptance to care across the sites. The last column displays data from the National Nursing Home Survey which describes the demographic characteristics of elderly persons over age 65 who were residing in nursing homes in 1985.

Examining these different demographic characteristics we find that the Living at Home sample is considerably older on average, (mean age 78), than in the general U.S. elderly population, but not quite as old as the Channeling clients and about five years younger than elderly nursing home residents who had a mean age of 83. It is important to note, however, that the median age of the Living at Home sample is 80. Indeed, if the sample is restricted to those 84 years and older, the Living at Home and Channeling samples are almost identical. However, both are still not as old as the nursing home sample, wherein 46% of elderly residents are over age 84.

The large percent of females (71%) targeted for care by both Living at Home and Channeling corresponds well to the 74% of elderly females receiving nursing home care. Far fewer individuals in both Living at Home and Channeling are married than is true for the general U.S. elderly population. However, the percent of individuals married in both Living at Home and Channeling is still considerably higher than is the case in the nursing home population. Both Living at Home and Channeling targeted a larger number of non-whites than are represented in the general U.S. population and included more non-whites than one would find in a nursing home population. Importantly, with respect to living arrangements, a majority (58%) of Living at Home clients lived alone. That is much higher than the comparable statistic for either the Supplement on Aging (32%) or the Channeling sample (37%). Median household income provides still another indicator of the vulnerability of the Living at Home sample, with $535 per month in median household income for the Living at Home sample compared to $649 (in 1988 dollars) for the Channeling group. Finally, regarding education, another consistent indicator of vulnerability, the majority (57%) of the Living at Home sample had less than a high school education.

Data on informal supports (not shown) indicate that 58% of LAHP clients had an available caregiver; however, only 64% of this group had either indefinite or short term (lasting one to six months) help available. The remaining 36% who reported a caregiver had help that was available only sporadically. The great majority of caregivers, not unexpectedly, were relatives of the client, with 76% of caregivers being either a spouse, sibling or child. Also, as expected, the great majority of caregivers (70%) were female.

Table 9 examines functional status of Living at Home clients, again comparing them whenever possible to similar characteristics for the Supplement on Aging and Channeling samples. With respect to cognitive status, Living at Home clients had a mean Mental Status Questionnaire (MSQ) error score of 2.7, indicating mild to moderate impairment. A score of five or more errors is considered to indicate severe impairment on this scale. Nineteen percent of the Living at Home sample fell into this category, compared to 34% of the Channeling sample. However, it is important to remember that Living at Home had a much higher percentage of individuals who live alone (58% vs. 37%, respectively). This difference in living arrangements probably explains the difference in severity of cognitive status impairment between these two samples, since it is very difficult for cognitively impaired individuals who live alone to be maintained in the community.

With respect to baseline health status, 18% of the Living at Home

TABLE 9. Functional Status: MSQ, IADL & ADL

(N = 959)

	MSQ	IADL	ADL
Mean Score	2.7, s.d.=3.2	3.9, s.d.=2.3	1.9, s.d.=2.4
No impairments		12	40
One impairment		8	16
Two impairments		9	15
Three or More impairments		71	29

sample had previously used a nursing home, a rate that is nine times higher than the general elderly population; 49% had been hospitalized in the past year, compared to 49% of the Channeling sample who were hospitalized in the last two months, indicating that the Channeling Demonstration population may have been more acutely ill than the Living at Home sample. Prevalence of poor vision was also higher in the Living at Home sample, about twice as high as it is in the general U.S. elderly population. With respect to the prevalence of other medical conditions, one to one correspondence was seen across all three samples with arthritis being the most common condition reported in all three, followed by high blood pressure or circulatory disease and heart disease.

Table 9 also indicates that, on average, LAHP clients had about four IADL impairments at baseline. Although 88% of LAHP clients had impairments in instrumental ADL, this is lower than the 99% found in the Channeling sample. The majority of LAHP clients (72%) were impaired in ability to travel independently in the community with the lowest number reporting impairment in ability to use the phone. On average, LAHP clients also had about two ADL dependencies at baseline. These are activities that clients either required some help with or were totally unable to do. This impairment score compares pretty well with the 2.7 mean ADL score of the Channeling sample, especially when one considers that no ADL screens were used for targeting. Examining the specific pattern of ADL impairments, we observed the customary pattern of hierarchical loss of function with the majority of clients (41%) being impaired in their ability to climb stairs compared to 10% who were impaired in their ability to eat.

Given the functional status and demographic characteristics of the Living at Home population, how do its service needs compare to those of other populations? Table 10 compares unmet service needs across the three different populations, and indicates that the general U.S. elderly population surveyed in the Supplement on Aging is much more likely to identify unmet needs for senior centers, special transportation and home nursing care. In the Living at Home group the number one unmet need was care coordination followed by help accessing benefits, need for comprehensive assessments and in-home services. The Channeling demonstration did not ask about

TABLE 10. Most Common Unmet Service Needs

SOA[a]	LAHP	CHANNELING[b]
1. Senior Center	1. Care Coordination	1. Housekeeping
2. Special Transportation	2. Help Accessing Benefits	2. Bathing
3. Home Nursing Care	3. Comprehensive Assessments	3. Meals
	4. Chore/Housekeeping	
	5. Homemaker	

a. 1984 Supplement on Aging, National Health Interview Survey, National Center for Health Statistics.
B. Applebaum, R. 1988 The Evaluation of the National Long Term Care Demonstration, Recruitment and Characteristics of Channeling Clients.

125

unmet needs in the area of care coordination or benefits but shows the same pattern of need for housekeeping, bathing, meals, which are all in-home supportive services. Thus, a noteworthy degree of correspondence in unmet needs is seen between numbers 1, 2, and 3 for Channeling, numbers 4 and 5 for Living at Home and number 3 for Supplement on Aging.

DISCUSSION

To summarize, we conclude from these data that Living at Home has successfully targeted a group of very frail seniors. The data demonstrate consistently that Living at Home has targeted a very old (median age 80) population that is poor, female, living alone and impaired in both instrumental ADLs and ADLs. This profile of LAHP clients is also fairly uniform, despite the lack of clear admission criteria and the great variability among the 20 sites. We conclude that this uniformity demonstrates a high degree of awareness on the part of providers about (1) the characteristics of the frail clients and (2) successful ways of identifying and enrolling them. Despite the lack of uniform targeting criteria across sites, the Lead Agencies seem to have succeeded in (1) communicating a profile of most vulnerable elderly to their staff and to the Affiliate service agencies in the networks and (2) targeting services to that group. Encouraging results have also been seen in the organizational change data, indicating that the networks were implementing more formal structural communication and coordination mechanisms as well as accessing important post-grant funding sources at the midpoint of the demonstration.

The next steps that we plan to take will include examining variability in client targeting across the sites to better understand its magnitude. Between now and the end of the evaluation (mid 1990), we will examine the service utilization data in order to examine variability in service use, controlling for baseline risk. In other words, we will examine whether there are any observable patterns in service utilization for particular groups of clients, categorized by degree of vulnerability. We will also examine, via the Time 3 organization change survey, the ability of the networks to remain intact and continue to provide service once Foundation funding ceases.

Together, these multiple types of data are anticipated to demonstrate whether voluntary health and social service networks that use existing benefits and entitlements can succeed in reducing unmet service needs while simultaneously tailoring services to unique local concerns. Factors which lead to successful efforts will be identified and assessed for potential replicability in other communities. The data can also be used to help define the ranges of community care users and service options that are possible across multiple community care sites. These data will be particularly useful to third party payors of community based care who are currently struggling to define eligibility criteria and the contents of service benefit packages.

REFERENCES

Applebaum, R. 1988. The Evaluation of the National Long Term Care Demonstration, Recruitment and Characteristics of Channeling Clients. *Health Services Research* 23(1): 51-66.

Binstock, R.H. 1987. Title III of the Older Americans Act: An analysis & proposal for the 1987 reauthorization. *The Gerontologist* 27(3): 259-65.

Louis Harris and Associates, Inc. 1982. Priorities and Expectations for Health and Living Circumstances: A Survey of the Elderly in Five English Speaking Countries. New York.

Hughes, Susan L. 1985. Apples and Oranges? A Review of Evaluations of Community-Based Long-Term Care. *Health Services Research* 20(4):261-287.

Hughes, Susan L. 1986. *Long Term Care: Options in an Expanding Market.* Rockville, MD: Aspen Publishers, Inc., Formerly Dow Jones Irwin.

Hughes, Susan L. and William G. Weissert. 1988. Living at Home. *Generations* 12:66-67.

Kemper, P., R. Applebaum and M. Harrigan. 1987. Community Care Demonstrations: What Have We Learned? *Health Care Financing Review* 8(4):87-99.

Kovar, M. and M. Chyba. 1984. Supplement on Aging, National Health Interview Survey, National Center for Health Statistics.

Weissert, William G. 1985. Estimating the Long-Term Care Population: Prevalence Rates and Selected Characteristics. *Health Care Financing Review* 6(4):8391.

Weissert, William G. 1985. Seven Reasons Why It Is So Difficult To Make Community-Based Long-Term Care Cost Effective. *Health Services Research* 20(4):423-433.

APPENDIX 1. Agencies Participating in LAHP National Demonstration

City	Agency Name
Boston, MA	South Cove Community Health Center
Buffalo, NY	University Hospital Home Medical Service
Charlotte, NC	Coordinated Care Management Corporation
Chicago, IL	Presbyterian Hospital
Cincinnati, OH	Council for Jewish Elderly
Denver, CO	Council on Aging of the Cincinnati Area
Durham, NC	Medical Care and Research Foundation
Miami, FL	Duke University Medical Center
Milwaukee, WI	Miami Jewish Home and Hospital for the Aged
Nashville, TN	Community Care Organizaton of Milwaukee County, Inc.
	Council of Community Services

New York, NY	East Harlem Council For Human Services, Inc.
	The New York Hospital-Cornell Medical Center
	St. Vincent's Hospital and Medical Center
Oklahoma City, OK	Areawide Aging Agency
Pasadena, CA	Huntington Memorial Hospital
Pittsburgh, PA	The Montefiore Hospital Association
San Francisco, CA	Northern California Presbyterian Homes
St. Paul, MN	Ramsey County Public Health Nursing Service
Tucson, AZ	Pima Council on Aging

Integrating the Frail and Well Elderly: The Experience of Senior Centers

Carole Cox
Abraham Monk

SUMMARY. This study examined the extent to which frail elderly are being integrated into multiservice senior centers in New York state. The data obtained from nearly 300 such centers indicates that directors agree in principle to accepting frail members but do not feel, in practice, they can handle more than 10 percent of their members being frail. They are more able to work with physically and sensorially impaired than with the mentally frail. Proper staff training and effective coordinative arrangements with other service agencies are good predictors of organizational capacity to integrate frail members.

SENIOR CENTERS AND THE WELL AGED

Senior centers are one of the earliest and largest forms of organized services specifically created for older persons in the United States. According to Lowy the number of older people actually participating in centers is 8 million, or one out of every three senior adults (1985). Projecting this figure into the future, by the year 2,000 it is estimated that there will be 32 million people over 65, and consequently, over 10 million possible center users. Yet the demand for senior centers may be substantially greater: the Harris poll found that almost 22 percent of those not currently attending a senior center would like to (Harris and Associates, 1981). When comparing users with non users profiles, repeated studies (Anderson, 1969; NCOA, 1972; NISC, 1974) have found that the latter group was more likely to experience serious health impediments. In

This study was supported by a grant from the AARP-Andrus Foundation.

the NCOA study, 22 percent of the nonmembers, versus 13 percent of the members had difficulty walking or climbing stairs. Moreover, nonusers were more likely to rate their health problems as "very serious."

Early centers were established primarily to counter the sense of isolation and loneliness that was likely to afflict many seniors, especially after the loss of a spouse, occupational roles, relocations, etc. Centers were therefore geared to enhancing socialization but invariably focused upon the activities of individuals expected to be able to manage for themselves (Maxwell, 1973). Centers thus became associated over the years with a well functioning and relatively younger cohort of older persons, and the goal of centers' programs was precisely the maintenance and prolongation of well being and self support among their members.

Earlier descriptions of senior center participants portray a population composed primarily of older, active and relatively healthy persons. They are mainly non-minority women (Pollack, 1970; Trela, 1971; Hansen et al., 1978; Ralston, 1984; Schneider et al., 1985). In only one study has frailness—as indicated by having mobility problems, being dependent on either a walker or crutches—been significantly associated with center participation (Ralston and Griggs, 1985).

However, since the establishment of the first senior centers in the 1940s there have been substantial demographic changes in the population of older persons. In 1940 the population group 65 and over comprised 6.8 percent of the U.S. population while by 1980 the proportion over 65 had increased to 11.3 percent and is predicted to exceed 13 percent by the year 2000 (U.S. Bureau of the Census, 1984). Moreover, the proportion of those 75 and over during the same period doubled proportionally from 1.7 percent to 3.4 percent with the 85 over population being the fastest growing age group in the country (U.S. Bureau of the Census, 1984).

These shifts in the population could imply that senior centers may no longer limit themselves to a predominantly "well" population which requires socialization enhancement only. Increased age is typically accompanied by increases in impairment and dependency and the need for more services. Whereas only 13 percent of noninstitutionalized persons 65 to 74 require functional assistance with activities, the proportion increases to 28% of those 75 to 84 and to 49% of those 85 and over (AARP, 1988).

SENIOR CENTERS AND THE FRAIL ELDERLY

The initial impetus for senior centers to reach out to the frail elderly came from Section 504 of the Rehabilitation Act of 1973 which became effective in 1977. This Act prohibits discrimination on the basis of handicap in any program or service receiving federal funds. The definition of "handicapped" includes hearing and visual losses and mobility impairments, conditions associated with aging and which may be ascribed to the frail. The Act further states that recipients of funds cannot deny qualified handicapped persons from participating in activities and that any special services for the handicapped, deemed necessary, must be as effective as those offered the non-handicapped.

This legislation, which provides a mandate for serving the frail elderly, was followed by the designation of senior centers as focal points for comprehensive delivery and coordination of community services and the emphasis, under the Older Americans Act Amendments of 1978, that services be directed towards those most in need.

The New York State Office for the Aging, in collaboration with the New York State Conference for the Aging, analyzed in 1981 the training and development needs of senior centers. The consensus was that senior centers were already serving a more frail and economically vulnerable population. They also identified the need for more programming and outreach to the vulnerable and minority elderly and for better clarification of the OAA legislative mandate to target services on the vulnerable elderly.

However, no state policy explicitly mandates the incorporation of frail elderly into senior centers. General incentives for providing services to the frail did evolve in some senior centers but resistances by staff to the incorporation of the high risk, frail elderly are often associated with the fear that it will jeopardize the affiliation and retention of the well aged who have been the traditional mainstays of the centers. They believe that centers have always been identified with wellness, not with infirmity, and that the frail will be better served in day care programs, nursing homes and homes for the aged. Moreover, it is argued that centers are not properly equipped to serve the very impaired, unless they change their entire programs and operational makeup. The question to be investigated is whether senior centers will remain specialized agencies for the "well" aged only or whether they may be counted as a legitimate resource in a battery of alternatives to institutionalization offered to the vulnerable aged.

RESEARCH OBJECTIVES

The main question addressed in this study is what role — if any — are senior centers, beginning to play in addressing the needs of the frail aged population.

The study was completed by the research staff of the Brookdale Institute on Aging and Adult Human Development at Columbia University, during the one year period that started on January 1, 1987, and focused on the ways in which the needs of the frail are being met by centers, as well as on the impact that this frail membership may have on other "well" users.

The next question has been whether it is feasible to adequately meet the needs of both the well and the frail elderly under one roof, in a single program context. At a time when federal resources are becoming more scarce but the older and more vulnerable population is increasing in numbers, the findings of this study may help to widen the range of services for larger segments of seniors, while making better use of service resources already in place.

METHODOLOGY

Data were collected through mail questionnaires sent to 282 senior center directors in New York State. The names of the centers, meeting the definition of a multipurpose senior center, were obtained through the New York State Office on Aging and the State's 56 Area Agencies on Aging. After three waves of questionnaires, responses were obtained from 198 directors thus reaching a 70 percent response rate.

In addition, site visits were conducted to 28 centers sampled throughout the state in order to collect in-depth information from their directors on the main questions guiding this study.

DESCRIPTION OF THE CENTERS

Preliminary fundings indicated that approximately half of the centers operated on budgets of less than $50,000 per year, not including funds for specific programs such as nutrition or the Retired Seniors Volunteers Program (RSVP). The primary source of center revenues were funds from the Area Agencies on Aging. The number of paid staff in the centers ranged in size from one to five persons, with a median staff of four. Centers also actively engaged volunteers in their programming, with a median of 15 volunteers per center. These volunteers were mostly involved in fundraising and transportation. Training of volunteers was minimal and generally consisted of only a general orientation to the center's programs.

The centers offered a wide range of services, with three of them: information and referral (87%), recreation and leisure (87%), and group meals (83%) being offered in almost all centers on a daily basis. Two-thirds of the centers (66%) also provided transportation although this was not necessarily targeted for the frail participants.

A majority had wheelchair ramps, handrails, extra wide hallways, and grab bars in bathrooms to assist the frail. Handrails were present, however, in less than one-third (32%) of the sites.

Center Participants

Center participants ranged in age, for the most part, between 65 and 84 years. Consistent with previous studies mentioned earlier, most were female and white. During the previous twelve month period, the number of center participants had increased in slightly more than half (52%) of the sites.

Only a small proportion of these participants, 10% were described by the directors as frail, and requiring some type of special assistance. Almost half of the directors (48%) felt that the 10 percent was the upper limit of frail that they could absorb into their programs, and slightly more than a quarter (27%) thought they could possibly accommodate as many as 20 percent. Perhaps because of these restrictive parameters, the proportion of frail in the centers tended to remain constant over the previous twelve months.

Over one-third of the frail participants were impaired due to hearing loss. This was followed by visual, memory, and mobility impairments. The directors felt that persons with these impairments were the easiest to integrate into their regular programs. The most difficult to integrate were persons with behavioral or emotional problems, or mental retardation. It is perhaps due to this difficulty that persons with these disabilities accounted for only 10 percent of the frail participants.

The Well Participants and the Frail

A primary focus of the study was the relationship between the well participants and the frail. Negative attitudes on the part of well elderly towards the impaired are not uncommon and can act as barriers towards integration. These attitudes may be particularly strong among the elderly who feel themselves at closer risk of many of the disabilities already afflicting their peers (Gozali, 1971).

However, the directors affirmed that the well were almost unanimously accepting (81%) of the frail, although they acknowledged that they were more accepting of friends and acquaintances who became frail, than of new participants who were already disabled at the time of joining the center. Reflective of the centers' ability to absorb specific types of impairments, the well members were also more accepting of the physical impairments, such as mobility, hearing, vision, and speech, than of persons with mental or emotional disabilities.

Many of the directors did attempt to counteract or change the resistant attitudes of the well. A slight majority of the centers (52%) utilized a "buddy" system in which well members are paired with frail persons. Discussions and films on particular impairments were used in almost half of the centers, while classes and sensitivity training were provided less frequently. Another strategy for fostering integration was to encourage the well to assist the frail with their meals, walking, and transportation.

The majority of the centers' staff (86%) were perceived by the directors as similarly accepting of the impaired, irrespective whether they were accepting old members who became frail or new members who were frail when they joined. The two primary difficulties experienced by the staff in working with the frail were a lack of time (63%) and inadequate training to meet specific needs (18%).

Programs for the Frail

A subtle distinction that emerges from this study is that merely accepting frail participants does not insure their integration into mainstream center programs, nor their actual blending with the rest of the membership. The latter seems to be a function of separate, specialized program targeted on the frail, and a favorable attitudinal climate among the well aged.

Very few of the centers—one out of six—had developed programs for persons with specific disabilities such as the hearing impaired or stroke victims (Table 1). In fact, it is unclear what the frail elderly did in the centers since they tended not to participate in the regular programs. Only 48% of the directors reported that the frail were involved in most of the formal activities.

A formal assessment of the capacity and ability of the impaired elderly to join in activities can provide a framework for encouraging integration. But, in only a minority of the centers (39%) were these assessments made on site. The assessments were, for the most part (64%), based upon the referrals from other agencies with only a small proportion (17%) using medical screenings. The absence of on-site assessments increases the risk that many of those who could possibly share in the regular activities are overlooked by the center staff.

Planning for the Frail

While most (80%) directors responded that they were interested in increasing the number of frail participants, less than a quarter (23%) actually had made plans for implementing such a program and only a third (35%) had actually increased the frail participants in the previous year. Over half of the centers (53%) did adopt a formal policy of acceptance of the frail elderly. Moreover, the majority of directors (75%) stated that they had made direct appeals to

Table 1

Programs and Planning for the Frail

Responses of Centers	Per Cent (n=197)
Specific programs for frail	9
Frail participate in most activities	4
On-site formal assessment	5
Assessments based on referrals	2
Medical screenings for assessments	10
Interested in increasing frail participants	1
Plans made for increasing frail	8
Increase in frail in previous 12 months	6
Trained staff for integration	7
Factors most essential for increasing frail	
Funds	3
More staff	11
Transportation	12
Facility improvements	13
Changes in participants' attitudes	14

the well participants to welcome them. However, few centers (34%) had actually trained their staff in strategies to facilitate their integration in ongoing programs.

In ranking the factors considered most essential for increasing the proportion of impaired elderly in the centers, the need for more funds was given top priority by 60% of the respondents. This was followed by "needs for more staff" (16%).

INTERAGENCY COOPERATION

Senior centers do not operate in isolation. They are part of a large network of community programs with whom links in planning and program coordination commonly occur (Krout, 1985). Many of these programs could potentially act both as referral sources and specialized service providers for the frail within the centers. However, most referrals to the senior centers came informally from relatives or friends. Very few referrals of the impaired originated from other community agencies.

There was some interagency coordination in working with the frail in the centers. Directors were most likely to receive program assistance from local health departments (55%), services for the visually (54%) and hearing (42%) impaired, hospitals (52%) and home health agencies (59%).

CONTINGENCY ANALYSIS

A contingency analysis was conducted to examine the relationship of specific factors relevant to integration, with the actual proportion of frail present in the centers. The proportion of frail in the centers was dichotomized at the median (10%) with centers categorized into two groups, those with less than 10% and those with more than 10% frail members.

The results of the analysis reveal that the size of the center budgets, although claimed to be most important to integration, did not actually influence the proportion of the frail in the centers, (Table 2) casting doubt on the key role played by funding. Furthermore, no relationship existed between having either a formal policy for incor-

Table 2

Relationships between Key Variables and Proportion of
Frail in Centers

	10% or Less (n=70)	11% or More (n=95)	Chi-Square
Budget			
Small	74.1	70.0	
Medium	18.5	22.9	n.s.
Large	7.4	7.1	
Change in Well Participants			
Increased	58.7	51.2	
Decreased	6.5	20.7	7.68*
Same	34.8	28.0	
Formal Policy			
In place	51.9	47.1	
No policy	48.1	52.9	n.s.
Programs for disabled			
Offered	22.9	14.3	
Not offered	77.1	85.7	n.s.

*p<.05

porating the frail elderly or having specific programs for them, and their actual participation in the centers.

An important finding did emerge in the relationship between the well and the frail. Although the directors had stated that the well were accepting of the impaired, the analysis indicated that those centers which increased the numbers of the frail in the previous year also experienced a significant drop in the number of well participants ($p < .05$). This suggests that the well elderly are not as tolerant of the frail as reported. In fact, their actual withdrawal from the centers negates any real integration.

MULTIVARIATE ANALYSIS

An analysis of variance showed no differences in the proportion of frail participants by either the types of physical supports in the centers or the size of the staff (Table 3). Both of these factors had been noted by the directors as essential prerequisites for increasing the number of frail members. The findings, however, reveal that these two factors may play a lesser role in the integration than originally claimed.

There was however, a strong positive association ($p < .001$) between the proportion of frail in the center and the number of agencies with which the centers coordinated their programs and obtained program resources. Unfortunately, it is not clear which came first, whether the increased number of frail facilitated links with other specialized agencies or if due to the more aggressive coordination, centers were able to expand the number of frail participants.

Equally important was the association between the number of frail and the number of trained staff at the centers ($p < .001$). Thus, although the size of the staff did not affect the proportion of impaired members, their quality or expertise, as suggested by their training did. Again, it is not known whether the training preceded or resulted from the increase in the number of frail participants.

A multiple regression analysis was conducted to determine the importance of selected independent variables, as predictors of the proportion of frail participants in a center. It revealed that having trained staff had the greatest impact on the proportion of frail (Table 4, B = .33), reinforcing the importance of the need for

Table 3

One-Way Analysis of Variance for Percentage of Frail and Key Variables

Key Variables	10% or Less	11% or More	Significance Level
Physical supports	6.0	6.6	n.s.
Coordinated service agencies	1.4	4.2	p<.001
Number of staff	3.5	4.1	n.s.
Number of trained staff	1.9	3.1	p<.001

Table 4

Multiple Regression Analysis for Proportion of Frail in Centers

Variables	Unstandardized beta	Standardized Beta
Budget	1.0	0.5
Staff	0.10	0.02
Volunteers	-0.22	-0.30**
Trained staff	3.0	0.33***

** p<.001
*** p<.0001

143

qualified staff. The results further substantiated that budget size and number of staff do not necessarily lead to greater integration. Most intriguing is the finding that the number of volunteers in a center was inversely related to the proportion of frail members. As frail participants could benefit from the additional assistance provided by volunteers, the reasons underlying this negative relationship merit further exploration.

The face-to-face interviews conducted with 28 center directors provided further information on the experiences and plans for integrating the frail into the centers' programs. While the mail surveys had shown the well members as not opposing the frail, the reverse was found in the interviews. The discussions with the directors supported the findings of the data analysis with regard to the resistance of the well elderly to letting the impaired into their programs. The core to the resistance appears to be the fear and threat of becoming frail themselves in the near future, with the result being that many of the well drop out of the centers.

Several directors also voiced concern about becoming "baby sitters" for nursing home patients. They did not have the facilities or staff to meet the needs of these persons. Conversely, many directors refused to use the label "frail" since by doing so staff would begin to differentiate between participants and the more impaired could potentially be left out of activities. Therefore, they sought to treat all participants as if no problem existed.

DISCUSSION

The primary question of this investigation was whether it is possible to meet the socialization and supportive needs of both the well and the frail aged within the framework of the thousands of multipurpose senior centers in the United States. Related to this question is the extent to which the frail are actually being integrated into the centers and the factors that facilitate or hinder such integration.

The findings suggest that the center directors can cope with a rather low percentage of no more than 10% of their members being frail. Furthermore, they are better able to integrate those with physical impairments than those with behavioral or emotional ones. At the same time, both the staff and the regular membership are more accepting of long standing participants who become progressively frail, than of strangers who are already frail when they join. Moreover, the decrease in the proportion of the well participants associated with the increase in the proportion of the frail suggests an overall reluctance towards integration which was confirmed in the face-to-face interviews.

Although the majority of the directors stated that they had formal guidelines for acceptance of the frail and were interested in increasing this group in the centers, only a minority had actually developed specific programs for incorporating them or for adjusting to their needs. There thus remains the question of what actually happens to the frail in the centers or how well their specific needs are being met. Acting as if no problem or difference exists may create the appearance of integration and participation while actually being a distancing form of program management that could be interpreted as insensitive and rejecting. The frail group may in fact remain isolated, or virtually segregated despite their formal enrollment in the centers.

Centers may sorely need better budgetary resources for implementing their overall programming. They may be right in their pleas for more and better staff. They may even build new facilities especially designed for the convenience of the frail. However, these factors alone would not automatically ensure a greater participation of this population. What appears to make the difference is, as stated above, the systematic training of the staff for working with this group and the coordination of these programs with other specialized agencies. Concentrating resources in these areas may be the most effective means to reaching the frail elderly.

Finally, what are the lessons derived from this study that could serve as recommendations for further action? At the risk of reiterating what has been already stressed in different parts of the text, four points need to be highlighted:

1. There can be no effective integration without systematic and in-depth training of both staff and volunteers, in all aspects pertaining to the needs of the frail.
2. Not all program activities are suitable for the frail. Their social

participation will actually be enhanced if offered differential programs that take into account their limitations.

3. Centers cannot do the job alone. They need to enlist an effective interagency network for obtaining specialized diagnostic, program, and service resources.

4. Centers must bring the issue to the attention of their mainstream well membership. Problems of resistances and negative attitudes must be examined, evaluated and dealt with in an amicable manner. Training is needed not only for the staff. The membership could similarly profit from a well designed and consistent educational program.

Center workers are aware that sociability and gregariousness cannot be mandated or legislated. Centers may try to be "frail-blind" and mix everybody in all activities, or they can selectively incorporate the frail in activities that are less demanding, or still offer specially adapted rehabilitative or supportive programs for those who cannot follow the pace of the mainstream membership. Centers can also act as an overall umbrella for an assortment of clubs or groups that respond to particular cultural, social or recreational interests. There is a risk that some of these clubs may end up exhibiting degrees of socioeconomic, educational or functional homogeneity that would virtually exclude the frail. Additional compensatory programs for the latter would then be in order.

There is no single programmatic formula. Many different paths may have to be tested in order to achieve the successful incorporation of all the elderly in senior centers.

REFERENCES

American Association of Retired Persons (1988) *A Profile of Older Americans,* Washington, DC: AARP Program Resources Department.

Anderson, N., (1969) "Senior Centers: Information from a Nationwide Survey," Minneapolis, Minnesota: American Rehabilitation Foundation.

Gozali, J., (1971) "The Relation Between Age and Attitudes toward Disabled Persons," *The Gerontologist,* 4, 289-291.

Hansen, A., Melma, H., Buckspan, L., Henderson, B., Helbig, B. and Fair, S. (1978) "Correlates of Senior Center Participation," *The Gerontologist,* 18, 193-199.

Harris, Louis and Associates, (1981) "The Myth and Reality of Aging in America," Washington, D.C.: The National Council on the Aging.

Krout, J. (1985) "Senior Center Linkages in the Community," *The Gerontologist*, 5, 510-515.

Lowy, L. (1985) "Multipurpose Senior Centers," in A. Monk (Ed.) *Handbook of Gerontological Services*, New York: Van Nostrand Reinhold, 274-301.

Maxwell, J., (1973) "Centers for Older People," Washington: National Council on the Aging.

National Council on the Aging, (1972) *The Multi-Purpose Senior Center: A Model Community Action Program*, Washington, D.C.: The Council.

National Institute of Senior Centers (1974) *Directory of Senior Centers and Clubs*, Washington, D.C.: National Council on the Aging.

Pollack, O. (1970) *Utilization Study of a Senior Citizen Center*, Philadelphia: Charles Weinsteing Geriatric Center.

Ralston, P. (1984) "Senior Center Utilization by Black Elderly Adults: Social Attitudinal and Knowledge Correlates," *Journal of Gerontology*, 39, 224-229.

Ralston, P. and Griggs, M. (1985) "Factors Affecting Utilization of Senior Centers: Race, Sex, and Socioeconomic Differences," *Journal of Gerontological Social Work*, 9(1), 99-111.

Schneider, M., Chapman, D., and Voth, D., (1985) "Senior Center Participation: A Two-Stage Approach to Impact Evaluation," *The Gerontologist*, 2, 194-200.

Trela, J. And Simms, L. (1971) "Health and Other Factors affecting Membership and Attrition in a Senior Center," *Journal of Gerontology*, 6, 46-51.

U.S. Bureau of the Census, (1984) *Demographic and Socio-economic Status of Aging in the United States*, Current Population Reports, Series P-23, N. 138, Washington, D.C.

Discharge Planning:
The Impact of Medicare's
Prospective Payment on Elderly Patients

Cynthia Stuen
Abraham Monk

SUMMARY. Discharge planning services have become very important to older adults who are subject to shortened hospital stays due to the prospective payment form of reimbursement based on diagnostic related groups (DRGs). A study of older adults discharged from three acute care hospitals in New York City shows a direct association between patients' satisfaction with their discharge plan and the number of services arranged by discharge planners. Patients told, "your DRGs are up" as the reason for their discharge, needed the greatest amount of help with activities of daily living. Implications for social workers offering discharge planning services are addressed.

BACKGROUND

The change from cost-based reimbursement to prospective payment for hospitalization represents the most significant change in the Medicare program since its inception in 1965, if disregarding the ill fated 1988 Medicare Catastrophic Amendments. Medicare benefits primarily affect adults aged 65 and over, the fastest growing segment of the U.S. population. Hence, the Prospective Payment System (PPS) is the first major fiscal experiment principally affecting older adults after almost two decades of policy stasis.

In 1983, the U.S. Congress approved a law (PL 98-21) which inaugurated a transition to PPS for hospital costs under the Medicare program. With the exception of four states already involved in cost-saving programs (New York, New Jersey, Maryland and Delaware), all acute care hospitals were subject to this new method of

149

reimbursement as of 1983. Under this new system, patients admitted to acute care hospitals are classified among 476 Diagnostic Related Groupings (DRGs) based on principal diagnosis, surgical procedures, additional diagnosis, age, sex and discharge disposition (Fetter, 1983).

This new procedure in Medicare reimbursement was placed into effect to curtail the rapidly escalating expenditures for hospitalization. The goal was to create an incentive for hospitals to contain the costs of treating a patient over the course of a hospital stay while maintaining an adequate level of quality and without restricting access to services for beneficiaries.

Many health and human service professionals, as well as, consumers and policymakers were concerned from the very inception of PPS that patients would end up being discharged 'quicker and sicker.' A study completed by the Hospital Association of Pennsylvania examined 4.5 million discharges from 244 community hospitals between 1982 and 1985. It showed a major decrease in average length of hospital stay and a concomitant increase in patient transfers to less costly care facilities such as nursing homes and rehabilitative facilities or to home care (Hospital Research Foundation, 1986). The average length of stay for all Medicare patients in short-stay hospitals decreased by 3.5 percent in fiscal year 1986, for a total decrease of 17 percent since the implementation of PPS (Guterman et al., 1988).

A preliminary study on the impact of PPS on long term care services, conducted by the U.S. General Accounting Office (1985), found that PPS creates a strong incentive for hospitals to shorten average length of stay even when patients' medical conditions warrant further need for care. In addition, Medicare enrollees are being admitted to various kinds of post-hospital care with more health deficits than prior to PPS, and with more extensive service needs (OTA, 1985, Bardsley et al., 1987). The demand for and the use of home health agency services has similarly expanded among Medicare beneficiaries in recent years (Phillips et al., 1987). True, this increase in utilization began prior to the institution of PPS but has grown at a rapid pace since. Utilization rates of skilled nursing facility services paralleled the growth of home health services following the implementation of PPS, after a period of relative stability from 1981 to 1983 (Guterman et al., 1988, U.S. Select Committee on Aging, 1989).

The PPS emphasis on cost containment places a renewed emphasis on proper discharge planning for older adults who are leaving hospitals sooner, and often in far greater need of skilled care. Families may be unprepared to cope, financial resources may be more difficult to obtain and community resources inadequate to meet the demands. Social workers and nurses, the two professions primarily involved in discharge planning, are under heavy pressure to get patients out of the hospitals as quickly as possible, while instructed they should not compromise the quality or continuity of care. While these mandates may be irreconcilable, they also may conflict with the needs of the patient and his or her family, ultimately placing the discharge planner under tremendous stress.

A study of the impact of PPS on discharge planners in New York City acute care hospitals revealed that tasks considered 'concrete,' e.g., screening patients for discharge, discussing discharge options, etc., are more frequently performed than 'softer' services, but no less essential, e.g., patient and family counseling (Stuen, 1987). This appeared to be a more radical change for social workers than nurses involved in discharge planning tasks.

STUDY OBJECTIVES

New York was not subject to the Prospective Payment System of reimbursement until January 1, 1986 due to an initial waiver. As a consequence, there was more time for speculation and debate about how the DRGs might affect Medicare-eligible patients. To a large extent this controversy centered on the fear that the elderly would be released prematurely with unsafe discharge plans, without adequate linkage to essential community support services and without proper monitoring of their post hospitalization plan of care. While much attention was being given to the impact of DRGs on hospital staff, the study reported here looked precisely at the impact of DRGs on the older adults discharged from acute care hospitals. Based on interviews with older adults, the study aimed to ascertain their: (a) understanding of their discharge plan, (b) satisfaction with the discharge plan, (c) knowledge of right to appeal discharge decisions, (d) preference for resources to meet their post hospitalization needs, and (e) perception of their health status.

The ultimate intent of this study was to provide health and social service practitioners, as well as policymakers with first hand information on how the Prospective Payment System is affecting older adults. It was hoped that its findings might help develop better community service resources and improve discharge planning practices.

METHODOLOGY

Sample

The data for this study were gathered from interviews with Medicare-eligible older adults who were discharged from three acute care hospitals in New York City: two were not-for-profit voluntary facilities and the third a city hospital. They will hence be designated as hospital A, B and C, respectively. In each of these institutions, discharge planning services were provided by the social services department.

Following orientation and training, hospital staff responsible for discharge planning services were asked to identify every older adult, those age 65 and over who had Medicare benefits, and who were ready for discharge. Each of these subjects was asked to give written consent to participate in the study. Such participation required the willingness to be available for an interview 4-5 weeks after discharge from the hospital. Participants were assured that any information they provided would be held confidential and that their identity would not be revealed. For patients unable to give consent, 'significant others' were approached. Reasons for refusal to participate were also documented. The original sample goal was seventy-five patients from each of the three participating hospitals. Copies of patient consent forms with addresses and telephone numbers were forwarded to the Columbia University Brookdale Institute on Aging.

Approximately three weeks after discharge from the hospital, patients were sent a letter reminding them of the study's purpose, thanking them for their agreement to be interviewed, and advising them to expect an interviewer's call. For subjects without a telephone, a personal appointment at their home was scheduled. If they were unable to keep the appointment, an enclosed post card could be returned or they were invited to call the Institute. In cases where the patient was not capable of being interviewed, significant others were sought.

Nine trained interviewers, primarily graduate students, completed interviews with subjects four to five weeks after discharge. Most interviews were conducted by telephone. The option of conducting the interview in Spanish was also available.

At the time of the interview, many participants were still convalescing. Consequently, the interviewers were not always able to gather the full information. One participating hospital served a large population of older adults residing in single room occupancy buildings where there were no telephones. Inadequate mail services made post discharge contacts there very difficult or impossible.

Variables

A series of demographic and descriptive questions about the living conditions and health condition of each patient were asked. Information was elicited about the length and total number of hospitalizations in the preceding year; the method whereby patients received a notice of discharge; the extent to which they knew about their right to appeal the hospital staff's decision; the nature of their discharge plan; the types of services arranged for and how satisfied they were with those services. Finally, self-reported health status was also queried, and a series of interviewer's perceptions of the interviewee were documented.

RESULTS

Profile of Participants

A total of 141 Medicare beneficiaries participated in this study. As noted, each was interviewed 4-5 weeks after their discharge from one of the three hospitals. Based on their responses to the survey instrument the following profile of participants can be drawn:

Age of the participants ranged from 55 to 96 years. The median and modal age were 76 and 78, respectively.

Forty-eight percent interviewed were widowed, 22% married, 5% divorced, 3% separated, and 22% never married. The majority of the participants were female (70%). Forty-six percent of the respondents had one or more children.

Seven out of ten or 74% of the respondents were White, 12.1% were Black, 10.7% Hispanic, 0.7% Asian and 2.1% other. A little more than half (53%) of the participants were Catholic, 24% Jewish, 20% Protestant, and 3% other.

Almost all, or 92% of the respondents were receiving Social Security benefits, 17.5% received additional aid from Supplementary Security Income (SSI), and almost 30% qualified for Medicaid. Forty-seven percent of the respondents received pensions from past employment, and 39% held private supplementary health insurance policies.

Living situations of the participants differed. Slightly more than half of the participants (N = 74, 54.8%) lived alone, while others lived with a spouse (N = 21, 15.6%), with a spouse and children (N = 8, 5.9%), with their children (N = 11, 8.1%), with relatives (N = 10, 7.4%), and with non-relatives (N = 7, 5.2%).

Nine (6.3%) respondents did not return home immediately after hospitalization. Five participants (3.5%) were admitted to nursing homes. The other four were admitted to various health related facilities.

At the time of the interview, most respondents (82.3%) perceived their current health to be fair or better: 39.4% fair, 27.7% good, 10.9% very good, and 4.3% excellent. Only 17.4% felt that their health was poor.

The median length of hospitalization was 16 days, while the modal length totaled 21 days. Although the majority of the respondents (80.9%) were not rehospitalized within the first month, the second stay was much shorter (median = 9 days, mode = 7 days), for those readmitted.

Patients' Satisfaction with Discharge Plan

One goal of this study was to identify whether the respondents were satisfied with the way their discharge was handled and whether they had knowledge of their right to appeal the plans the hospital had made for them.

In the majority of cases (77.3%), a physician was the first person to tell a respondent that they were ready to leave the hospital. Nurses or social workers informed the patients of discharge plans in only 8% of the cases.

At the time of discharge, 85.6% of the participants were told that they were medically ready to leave the hospital, or that they no longer needed to stay in the hospital. The other portion of the group, 14.4%, were told that their "DRGs were up" or that "Medicare won't cover you anymore." Only 7.9% of the participants recalled being given written notification of their discharge. At the time of the interview, only 33.6% of the participants were aware of their right to appeal the discharge plans made by the hospital.

The majority of the patients and/or family members (70.2%) received some assistance from the hospital in making their discharge plans, and 35.3% of the patients were directly involved in developing these plans. Overall, the participants (89.9%) were satisfied with their discharge plans and with the post-hospital care they continued receiving (85.9%). It included skilled nursing care, homemaker services, home attendant, physical therapy, speech therapy, occupational therapy, day care, meals on wheels, transportation to and from hospital clinics and equipment rental. On the average, two discharge services were arranged for each patient. Three of the most frequently utilized services were in-home nursing (56.9%), transportation (36.9%), and equipment rental (33.1%).

Although only 10% of the participants were dissatisfied with their discharge plans, a profile of this group was developed in order to document any gaps in the current service delivery system and to guide the planning of future services. About two thirds of those who were dissatisfied, (63.6%) indicated that they were not involved in arranging their discharge plans. More than half (54.5%) were not aware of their right to appeal the hospital's discharge decisions, and again, nearly two thirds, (63.3%) felt that they were not ready to leave the hospital. For this last group, little or no post-hospital services were arranged for them by the hospital. At the time of the interview, 60% felt that they were in poor health. Nearly three quarters of this group lived alone and over half did not have children. These dissatisfied participants, were readmitted to the hospital at the same rate as those who were satisfied; however, nearly half (45.5%) of them needed the most help with the activities of daily living.

The participants' satisfaction with their discharge plans was found to be related to the specific services which were rendered to them after their discharge. In fact, many of the patients who were satisfied were still receiving post-hospital services at the time of the survey interview, approximately 4 to 5 weeks after their hospitalization. Furthermore, the number of services required and arranged for each of the participants did not appear to be related to their diagnosis at the time of their initial admission or readmission, their living situation or the presence of their children.

The Impact of DRGs

The vast majority of the subjects, (89.4%) were told that they were medically ready to leave the hospital. However, when compiling a profile of those who were informed that their "DRGs were up" or that "Medicare won't cover you anymore," it was found that a statistically significant number of the respondents in this category (61.5%, $F = 19.27$, $p < .000$) felt they were not ready to leave the hospital. Whether these participants were discharged before they were truly physically ready or whether the hospital was medically justified is difficult to assess. Of those who were told that they were medically ready to leave, 20% were soon readmitted. The rate of readmission among those participants who were told in one way or another that their "DRGs were up," was slightly higher, 30%. This relationship is not statistically significant given that only a small number of the respondents were told that Medicare would no longer cover their services. It is interesting to note however that a higher percentage (46.2%) of this sub-group (those told their DRGs were up) were initially admitted with chronic diagnoses, in comparison to the total group (38.7%). Although no one in this subgroup felt that they were in excellent health, the majority, 61.5%, felt in fair health, 23.1% in good health and only 15.4% felt they were in poor health.

This subgroup did not appear to differ from the total group of participants in terms of racial or ethnic composition, or their living situation. The majority lived alone (69.2%), 7.7% resided with a spouse and a child, and 15.4% resided with children. No one in this group resided with only a spouse. The group was evenly divided between those with children and those without any children.

Much like the rest of the population under study, they were satisfied with the post-hospital services they had been receiving at the time of the interview. It is important to note that 66.7% of these participants who were told their "DRGs were up," needed the greatest amount of help with the activities of daily living.

Not surprisingly, the average length of stay among those who were told that their "DRGs were up" or "Medicare won't cover you any more" was longer (53.4 days) than those who were told that they were medically ready to leave the hospital (25.1 days).

Patients' Post-Hospitalization Status

Although the majority of the respondents had not been readmitted at the time of their interview in this study, a profile of those rehospitalized was compiled. In order to study this group in greater detail, the scales of personal activities of daily living and instrumental activities were computed for all participants. They were drawn from the Multidimensional Functional Assessment: the OARS Methodology (Pfeiffer, 1976).

Participants were asked to rate 16 activities in terms of the difficulty they presented to them. They used the following scale: "1 = do it yourself easily; 2 = do it yourself, but it's not easy; 3 = do it only if someone helps; 4 = cannot do it even with help." For the purpose of analysis, each individual's responses were added. Then, the respondents were divided into three equal groups according to their degree of limitation: 16-28, needing the least assistance; 29-41 needing limited assistance; 42-64, needing the most assistance. This scale was significantly associated to the respondents self-reported health, ($F = 24.16$, $p < .002$). Predictably those in the poor health group needed the most assistance with activities of daily living, and the opposite was true for those in good health. The activities of daily living scale was also statistically significant for persons who were told that their "DRGs were up," ($F = 7.204$, p. < .027). Of those who required the least amount of help, only 3.7% were told that Medicare would no longer pay for their hospital stay. However, 28.6% of those requiring the most amount of help were told that their "DRGs were up" (see Table I).

Comparison of the Three Hospitals

Although there were no apparent demographic differences in the respondent population among the three hospitals, variations did emerge in terms of discharge planning services. As mentioned in a previous section, 70.2% of the participants received assistance in planning for their post-hospital care. Of these hospital A was more than twice as likely to have arranged some type of discharge plan than hospitals B or C. This difference proved to be statistically significant at the $p < .000$ level. As noted in Table II, 50.5% of discharge plans made for every participant were completed by hospital A, while hospitals B and C each arranged only 27% and 22% respectively of the plans in question.

When analyzing the variability in total services received by the participants, significantly more services were reported arranged by hospital A at the time of discharge than hospital B or C ($F = 12.1$, $p < .000$). On the average, hospital A arranged three services per patient, in contrast to an average of one service by the other two hospitals. Consequently, hospital A arranged more transportation services than hospital B or C (Chi Square-12.77, $p < .001$). However, it is important to note that there were no significantly different inpatient services rendered to patients with similar diagnosis at any of the three hospitals.

In addition, analysis of this survey's data indicates that there is a direct association between patients' satisfaction with their discharge plans, and the number of services arranged by the hospital for their post-hospitalization. Of the participants who were satisfied with their discharge plans, 53% of the patients were discharged from Hospital A in comparison to 28% from Hospital B and 19% from

TABLE I

ACTIVITIES OF DAILY LIVING VARIABLES

	A. Need Least Help (Scores 16-28)	B. Need Some Help (Scores 29-41)	C. Need Most Help (Scores 42-64)
Patients told "DRGs are up" or "Medicare will no longer cover"............	3.7%	11.1%	28.6%
Satisfied with services they are receiving.......	9.3%	90.6%	86.1%
Admitted with acute diagnosis.................	58.3%	61.4%	66.7%
Admitted with chronic diagnosis.................	41.7%	38.6%	33.3%
Readmitted to hospital...	7.5%	23.3%	26.2%
Services arranged at discharge.................	21.0%	14.0%	16.0%
Perceived health:			
Excellent.............	12.8%	0.0%	2.4%
Very good.............	17.9%	11.6%	4.9%
Good.................	35.9%	34.9%	14.6%
Fair.................	25.6%	39.5%	46.3%
Poor.................	7.7%	14.0%	31.7%

159

TABLE II

PATIENT SATISFACTION WITH DISCHARGE PLANNING

PATIENT REPORTED HOSPITAL ARRANGED DISCHARGE

	Hospital A (N=56)	Hospital B (N=53)	Hospital C (N=32)	Total
Yes	50.5	27.3	22.2	100%
No	11.1	66.7	22.2	100%

(P<.000)

PATIENT SATISFIED WITH DISCHARGE

	Hospital A (N=56)	Hospital B (N=53)	Hospital C (N=32)	Total
Yes	53.1	27.6	19.4	100%
No	0.0	54.5	45.5	100%

(P<.003)

PATIENT SATISFIED WITH SERVICES

	Hospital A (N=56)	Hospital B (N=53)	Hospital C (N=32)	Total
Yes	51.8	28.2	20.2	100%
No	7.1	57.1	35.7	100%

(P<.007)

Hospital C. (This difference was statistically significant at the p < .003 level.) Also, an analysis of variance conducted showed a significant association between satisfaction and services rendered (F = 10.12, p < .007) (see Table II).

DISCUSSION OF FINDINGS

This study found that most patients, particularly those with acute conditions, were satisfied with the hospital in-patient services, their discharge plans, and the post-hospital care they received. Study data also indicate that patients' dissatisfaction was not a valid predictor of readmittance. However, it is interesting to note that a sizeable group of those respondents who were dissatisfied with services received in or out of the hospital, suffered from chronic conditions. Because hospitals are predominantly focused on acute care, they do not seem prepared to handle and can ill afford to provide the continuous care these patients need. Reclassification of acute care beds to 'alternate level of care' beds has been one response among many New York City hospitals. Ultimately, while the hospitals were legally correct in saying, "Your DRGs are up," as a reason for discharge, they were far from meeting both the patients' medical and emotional needs.

Those who suffer from chronic conditions tend to be more dependent than those afflicted with acute illnesses. This is evident from the high number of ADL supports these patients received after hospitalization. Hence, without comprehensive post-hospital care arranged for them, these patients were likely to feel neglected in their care.

Hospitals can reduce such feelings by placing a greater emphasis on linking patients to community-based services equipped to meet their long term care needs. This study indicates that hospital A did in fact make a greater effort to provide such linkage, and as a result, a higher percentage of their patients stated they were satisfied. Hospitals B and C may have tried to place patients in community-based settings, but given the fact that they serve a lower income population, and since most community-based care, such as home care, is largely paid out-of-pocket, it is conceivable that these patients were simply not able to afford the service.

In 1987, the State of New York passed legislation aimed at protecting all patients, regardless of age or income, from being discharged before they were medically ready. The New York State law, which became effective January 1, 1988, requires that hospitals provide each patient with a written notification of discharge and assures patients of their right to appeal for an independent review. Only 7.9% of the participants of this study recall receiving such a notification of their discharge. It ought to be noted that this study was conducted prior to the law going into effect. It is conceivable that the results would have been more positive had the study been conducted after the passing of the State law.

Overall, this study's findings corroborate other national surveys which conclude that most hospitals are doing reasonably well in adapting to the goals of the Prospective Payment System. They are doing better, as stated, with conditions requiring acute care.

IMPLICATIONS FOR SOCIAL WORK

Discharge planning has an uneven history in social work practice. When medical social work was begun in 1905 by Dr. Cabot, its principal function was to help in post-hospital planning so patients could sustain their health gains.

Social workers who focused on the 'mind' of the patient as the primary mode of intervention began to separate themselves from the medical social workers in 1926. Psychiatric social workers were rebutted by medical social workers with claims that they too were concerned with the emotional needs of their patients. In many settings, discharge planning came to be relegated to social work paraprofessionals because it was assumed it required less knowledge and skill than the counseling function (Germain, 1984). Yet many social workers began recognizing the complexity of the discharge function and concomitantly, the clinical expertise required to resolve conflicts between family members and health care personnel, on the one hand, and to reduce emotional stress suffered by the patient while being discharged, on the other (Regensberg, 1978).

Even prior to implementation of PPS, discharge planning occupied a great deal of a social worker's time in acute care hospitals (Lurie et al., 1981). The American Hospital Association surveyed its membership and identified hospitals offering services specifically for older adults. Those hospitals (N = 689) reported that discharge planning was the most frequently offered social service (75%) with the next highest (47.6%) reported as information and referral (Evashwick et al., 1985).

Public Law 99-509 amended the Social Security Act to require hospitals to provide patients with a notice of hospital discharge rights upon admission, and to have a discharge planning program as a condition of Medicare participation (Omnibus Budget Reconciliation Act of 1986, Section 9305). The Joint Commission on Accreditation of Hospitals has issued special guidelines recognizing discharge planning as part of higher quality service. The American Hospital Association has also approved guidelines for discharge planning and defines discharge planning as an interdisciplinary hospital-wide process that should be available to aid patients and their families in developing a feasible post-hospital plan of care.

The social work profession today appears to be reemphasizing discharge planning as it becomes an increasingly important component of hospital management and operation (Blazyk and Canavan, 1985). Social workers are redefining and regaining discharge planning functions that many of them relinquished, primarily to nurses, in the past. Bailis (1985) suggests social workers have not been aware that discharge planning offers a stronger potential *raison d'etre* for social work departments than psychotherapy. PPS, according to some leaders in this field, provides an opportunity for social workers to upgrade their functions and status, given that the proper discharge of patients is of the utmost importance to hospitals for their fiscal survival (Coulton, 1984; Kane, 1983; Reamer, 1985).

The nursing profession has also staked a claim to the provision of discharge planning, and many nurses believe that they are better suited to discharge planning because they can perform physical assessments, as well as insure continuity of care while the patient is still in the hospital (Dake, 1981). There is no denying that a nurse's input is critical in the discharge planning process with older adults, and social workers should welcome their partnership, in a multidisciplinary team.

Fitzig (1988 p. 6) aptly states "The realization that no single profession has the knowledge and skill to respond completely to the many problems presented by an individual or family makes the discharge planning process a natural for an interdisciplinary approach . . . it doesn't really matter who controls or coordinates the process as long as it is comprehensive and meets patients needs." Major fiscal experiments such as PPS provide a real challenge to all health professionals to address individual needs while recognizing organizational needs for financial survival.

REFERENCES

Bailis, S.S., A Case for Generic Social Work in Health Settings. *Social Work*, 30(3), 209-213, (1985).

Bardsley, M., Coles, J. and Jenkins, L., *DRG's and Health Care*, King's Publishing Office: London, (1987).

Blazyk, S. and Canavan, M.M., Therapeutic Aspects of Discharge Planning. *Social Work*, 30(6), 489-496, (1985).

Coulton, C.J., Confronting Prespective Payment: Requirements for an Information System. *Health and Social Work*, 9(1), 13-24, (1984).

Dake, W., Nursing Responsibilities for Discharge Planning in a Community Hospital. *Quality Review Bulletin*, October, 26-31, (1981).

Evashwick, C.J., Rundell, T., and Goldiamond, B., Hospital Services for Older Adults. *The Gerontologist*, 25(6), 631-637, (1985).

Fetter, R.B., The New ICD-9-CM Diagnosis-related Classification Scheme. Health Care Financing Administration, Baltimore, Md., U.S. Dept. of Health and Human Services, (1983).

Fitzig, C., Discharge Planning: Nursing Focus in *Discharge Planning: An Interdisciplinary Approach to Continuity of Care*. National Health Publishing, Owings Mills, Md. (1988).

Germain, C.B., *Social Work Practice in Health Care: An Ecological Perspective*. The Free Press, New York, (1984).

Guterman, S., Eggers, P.W., Riley, G., Green, R.F., and Terrell, S.A., The First Three Years of Medicare Prospective Payment: An Overview. *Health Care Financing Review*. Vol. 9, No. 3, 66-77, (1988).

Hospital Research Foundation, Utilization Patterns in Pennsylvania's Hospitals: Aggregate Data by Pay or Class. Philadelphia, PA. (1986).

Kane, R.A., Minding Our PPO's and DRG's. *Health and Social Work*, 8, 82-84, (1983).

Lurie, A., Pinsky, S. and Tuzman, L., Training Social Workers for Discharge Planning. *Health and Social Work*, 6(4), 12-18, (1981).

Pfeiffer, E., *Multidimensional Functional Assessment: The OARS Methodology*. Duke University, Center for the Study of Aging and Human Development: Durham, N.C. (1976).

Phillips, E.K., Fisher, M.E., MacMillan-Scattergood, D., Baglioni, Jr., A.J. and Torner, J.C., Home Health Care: Who's Where? *Journal of Public Health*, 77(6), 733-734, (1987).

Reamer, F.G., Facing Up to the Challenge of DRGs, *Health and Social Work*, 10(2), 85-94, (1985).

Regensberg, J. *Towards Education for Health Professions*, Harper and Row, New York, (1978).

Stuen, C., Prospective Payments and Hospital Discharge Planners Roles, *Doctoral Dissertation*, Columbia University, NY. (1987).

U.S. General Accounting Office, Information Requirements for Evaluating the Impacts of Medicare Prospective Payment on Post-hospital Long-Term Care Services: Preliminary Report. (Report to Senator John Heinz) GAO/PEMD-85-8, February 21 (1985).

U.S. Office of Technology Assessment, Medicare's Prospective Payment System: Strategies for Evaluating Cost, Quality and Medical Technology. OTA-H-262, Washington, DC: U.S. Government Printing Office, October (1985).

U.S. Select Committee on Aging, Health Care Costs for America's Elderly, 1977-78, No. 101-712. U.S. Government Printing Office, Washington, DC, March (1989).

... ...
... ...
... ...

Adult Day Care Services
for the Elderly and Their Families:
Lessons from the Pennsylvania Experience

Lenard W. Kaye
Patricia M. Kirwin

SUMMARY. This paper summarizes the findings of a statewide evaluation of adult day care centers in Pennsylvania. It concludes that these centers perform a much needed respite and socialization function. As demand for adult day care continues growing, there is need to establish quality care standards, improve transportation and add counseling services for both the clients and their caregivers.

This paper presents an overview of adult day care (ADC) programs with particular attention given to the assessment of participants' need, service utilization patterns, and the potential benefits to be derived from this noninstitutional interventive strategy. The function of social work practice in ADC is also considered and, finally, recommendations for program planning and development are offered. Findings from a statewide evaluation of ADC in the Commonwealth of Pennsylvania provide the basis for this analysis (Kaye and Kirwin, 1989).

BACKGROUND

Adult day care for the elderly is an integrated concept in community care systems originating in England, having evolved from the

The research on which this paper is based was produced with funds provided under Contract No. 871003 from the Pennsylvania Department of Aging.

geriatric psychiatric concept of comprehensive care developed in the Soviet Union (McCuan and Elliott, 1977; Padula, 1983). The first program in the United States similar to geriatric day care in England began in 1947 under the auspices of the Menninger Clinic (Adult Day Care, 1983; Mehta, 1975).

In 1978, an official federal directory identified nearly 300 ADC programs in 40 states serving more than 5,000 persons. In 1989, over 2,000 centers were operational in all 50 states serving more than 70,000 older adults. Forty-four states have developed state standards for licensure, funding, or certification (Von Behren, 1989).

While this rapid growth is, in part, a reflection of escalating interest in the development of long-term care alternatives in the community, it is significant that these programs developed despite the absence of any national policy to support this concept and without a permanent funding base. "The growth of ADC has truly been a grass-roots effort, arising out of the concern of local communities for the quality of life and the care of their elders" (Crossman, 1987, p. 3).

Hooyman (1986) described two overall purposes of ADC initiatives to be: (1) the provision of meaningful activities for the older adult; and (2) the availability of respite for families of frail elders. There is, however, a lack of clarity of program goals. For example, Kane and Kane (1987) have pointed out that day care is sometimes expected to improve or maintain overall functioning in the program participant, while at other times it is expected to enhance social involvement or alleviate depression. Respite for caregivers is also a goal often allowing a family member to remain employed.

Wilson indicated that ADC centers assist impaired older people in maintaining their usual place of residence, thereby avoiding the possibility of institutionalization (1984). Ohnsorg (1981) supports Wilson's assertion that all ADC programs "have a common denominator: to provide a noninstitutionalized support system for persons who otherwise have difficulty in maintaining independent living status in the community setting" (p. 18). Adult day care has been similarly defined as a community-based group program designed to meet the needs of functionally impaired adults through an individual plan of care. It is structured and comprehensive, providing health, social, and related support in a protective setting during any part of a day, but less than 24-hour care. (Von Behren, 1989, p. 14)

Indeed, John Melcher (D-Montana), past Chairman of the Senate Special Committee on Aging called day care "a more humane and cost-effective alternative to nursing homes and hospitals" (April 18, 1988).

As Kay Larmer, Chair of the National Institute on Adult Day Care (1988) has pointed out, at an average cost of $31 for 6 to 8 hours of client care and caregiver respite, adult day care is less costly than paid care in the home at $8-$10 per hour, or residency in a skilled nursing home at $68-$100 per day. Therefore, day care services may provide new hope in addressing some of the problems of the elderly. Yet, in the absence of an overarching national policy, an uncoordinated variety of sources fund variant models of day care services (Bilitski, 1985).

In reviewing previous programmatic studies, Harder et al. (1983) concluded that while the benefits of the program are demonstrable, and ADC may indeed prolong lives, it has not saved money. The critical policy issue is, how much is this service worth? Unfortunately, criteria on which to base this value decision, have not been defined.

Stassen and Holahan (1981) suggested that: (1) ADC generally enhanced and affected positive participant outcomes; (2) ADC did not appear to have affected inpatient hospital service utilization; (3) to a very limited extent, ADC substituted for nursing home care and some ambulatory services; and (4) ADC appeared to increase the total cost of care, as many people who normally would not have skilled or intermediate care, were using ADC.

Nonetheless, despite the possibility of increased costs, ADC and other community-based programs may enhance well-being and therefore be more desirable. According to Stassen and Holahan, this is the most persuasive reason for day care programs (1981).

These authors reported a reduction in mortality, increased cognitive functioning, heightened social activity, and high levels of client satisfaction as reported in several studies (Weissert, 1977; Weissert et al., 1979; Arling and Romaniuk, 1982; and Bilitski, 1985). On the other hand, no clear improvements in functional ability have been documented (Weissert, 1977; Weissert et al., 1979).

As Rhodes (1982) has noted:

> Adult day care is based on the premise that the elderly maintain their mental and physical wellbeing longer and at higher levels of functioning in the community and home-integrated milieu as opposed to institutional settings. Support services are geared to maintaining and stabilizing the elder to prevent premature institutionalization. (pp. 1-2)

In addition to controversies regarding the potential cost-savings of this program intervention, further controversy evolved from early advocates of the rather disparate medical and social program models in ADC (Aaronson, 1983; Koenen, 1980; Weissert, 1976). However, it is acknowledged today that the distinctions between day health and social day care are blurred (Kane and Kane, 1987; Von Behren, 1989), and ADC is regarded by the latter author as a generic label for all types of program regardless of the population served, the range of services, or funding sources.

ADC IN PENNSYLVANIA

ADC centers began operations in Pennsylvania during the late 1960s and early 1970s. In the 1980s several evaluation efforts (Bilitski, 1982, 1983, and 1985; Kirwin, 1986, 1988, 1989; Rhodes, 1982) noted increased client satisfaction and successful senior center program integration, as well as a higher incidence of dementia among program participants than in earlier studies (Weissert, 1975; Weissert, 1977).

Kirwin (1988), reporting on an analysis of three suburban Philadelphia county adult day care programs (N = 64), supported previous studies which indicated a low use of services by the multi-impaired elderly (Smyer, 1980). This was true even for the multi-impaired who had been attending ADC programs for over 17 months, and was especially the case for those individuals with intact informal support systems and the absence of a history of mental illness.

AN EVALUATION OF ADC IN PENNSYLVANIA

Much of the data presented in this paper are drawn from an evaluation of area agencies on aging (AAA)-funded ADC programs in the Commonwealth of Pennsylvania. This state-wide analysis aimed to better understand the characteristics and needs of persons receiving ADC in Pennsylvania during the period 1986-87.

Completed in 1989, this study specifically inquired about the socio-economic and functional characteristics of service recipients, their reasons for service utilization, their met and unmet needs and their informal caregivers, facilitators and barriers to service delivery, significant funding sources and component costs of service provision, staffing patterns and activity schedules, patterns of service utilization, assessment procedures, reasons for termination, and benefits derived from participation.

Mail survey questionnaires and in-person field interviews served as the primary methods of data collection. Secondary data were collected from a 25% random sample of client records (N = 290) maintained by area agencies on aging in 11 counties varying in terms of their geographic location, size of their 60 years and over population, and type of program funding (program vs. client funded services).

Primary data were collected by means of face-to-face structured interviews with elder ADC clients (N = 54) and their family caregivers (N = 67). Structured mail questionnaires were completed by ADC program directors (N = 59) and area agency on aging program managers (N = 26). An advisory committee comprised of area agency on aging and ADC organization representatives as well as gerontological scholars was convened. This group critiqued draft versions of the survey instruments (Time 1) and participated in the interpretation of study findings (Time 2). Study instrumentation included original and previously developed indices gauging: functional capacity; life satisfaction; mental, physical, and emotional health; and service provision levels.

Findings derived from the Pennsylvania study in combination with a comparative analysis of previously conducted state and national ADC research served as the major data sources for the presentation of information to follow.

THE NEED FOR ADC

Data from this study suggest that there is general consensus concerning why clients utilize ADC services. From the family caregiver's perspective, five reasons for utilization stand out: (1) socialization for the client; (2) respite for the caregiver; (3) increasing client contentment; (4) maximizing the client's functional capacity; and (5) providing respite for the client. It is interesting to note that the family caregiver perceives ADC as serving a respite function for both the family caregiver and the elder. Interviewed clients most frequently mentioned socialization (67% of the time) as the reason ADC services were used. Family caregivers less frequently pointed to the potential contributions of ADC as a source for rehabilitation of the client and as an alternative to institutionalization.

It is interesting to note that female family caregivers — these were usually wives and daughters — were more likely than men to use ADC as an "alternative to institutionalization" (e.g., nursing home placement) (t = 2.18, p < .05). Furthermore, as might be expected, employed caregivers were significantly more likely to list "client respite" (t = 2.56, p < .01) or "caregiver respite" (t = −3.15, p < .001) as reasons for utilization than nonworking caregivers. And, caregiver stress was found to be greatest among employed family members who cared for mentally impaired elders.

A review of the client files concerning the bases for initial requests for ADC services in Pennsylvania reaffirm the importance of the respite function. More than 55%, or 160 cases, indicated needed relief for caregivers as the basis for application for service. These files indicated that the most common referral source for an ADC applicant was the relative of the older adult. This was the case 38% of the time. Community agencies and programs were identified as referral sources less frequently (30% of the time).

THE ASSESSMENT PROCESS IN ADC

Once the client locates ADC services, the agency performs an assessment of eligibility. In the case of AAA-funded ADC, this assessment may be completed by a staff person at the ADC program and/or by a representative of the AAA. More often than not, ADC staff do their own reassessment of the client rather than an AAA case manager.

The main eligibility criterion for admission to ADC services is the applicant's physical and mental status. In the case of AAA-funded programs, age is the next most important criterion. Less frequently considered criteria include the status of an applicant's informal support network, their level of financial need, and the quality of the match between the older adult and the client population served by a particular ADC program.

Information collected during the ADC assessment may include:

a. Source of referral
b. Basis for initial service request
c. Demographic data (e.g., age, sex, ethnicity, household composition, size of household, marital status, caregiver employment status, living arrangements, extent of social supports)
d. Physical health status
e. ADL capacity
f. Social participation levels
g. Self sufficiency levels
h. Emotional status
i. Intellectual functioning levels
j. Financial status

Reassessments are commonly performed every three to six months and allow for the charting of changes in the service recipient's status in the various areas outlined above.

THE TYPICAL CONSUMER OF ADC SERVICES

In 1985, the National Institute of Adult Daycare, a membership unit of the National Council on the Aging, Inc., conducted a national survey of ADC programs. An in-depth analysis of these data was performed by Von Behren (1988). It revealed that nationally, the participant mean age was 72.9. Income averaged $483.45 a month. Nearly 19% of program recipients lived alone in independent housing, while another 12% lived on their own in congregate housing. Sixty-four percent lived with a spouse, relative, or friend. Seven percent of these elders were found to be incontinent; 18% were cognitively impaired and needed constant supervision (Von Behren, 1988). Adult day care participants in this national study attended ADC programs, on the average, 3 days a week (Von Behren, 1989).

The typical ADC service recipient in the Pennsylvania evaluation did not vary substantially from those consumers profiled in the national study. The typical Pennsylvania ADC client was a 77 year old, white female, living with a daughter or spouse in a single family dwelling and needing assistance with at least three physical activities of daily living and five or more instrumental activities of daily living. The greatest degree of physical impairment was registered by those clients with Alzheimer's disease, cardio-vascular problems, and to a lesser degree, depression and blindness. Elder recipients of service had a median monthly income of $481 and were usually dependent on a single source of income (Social Security). Generally, clients attended ADC 3 days a week, and 6 hours a day.

SERVICE UTILIZATION PATTERNS IN ADC

What specific services are provided by ADC programs? Are these services provided by program staff or are they received through a contractual arrangement with an outside party?

National survey data (Von Behren, 1989) document ADC centers providing just over two of the following professional services: nursing, social services, physical therapy, and occupational therapy. For those ADC programs with a medical emphasis, the average was almost one of the following: physician assessment; physician treatment; psychiatry; podiatry; or dentistry.

In order to assess the frequency with which particular services were provided to ADC clients in the Pennsylvania study, the study questionnaire completed by ADC directors included a Service Provision Index (SPI) previously developed by Kaye (1982). The SPI contains 19 services delivered with varying frequency by community service programs for the elderly such as shopping, recreational activities, personal care, home repairs, etc. The alpha, a measure of internal reliability, was .70 for the SPI indicating a moderate level of internal reliability. As seen in Table 1, ADC programs reported providing a variety of services with some frequency (Mean = 2.74, S.D. = .54). The score range for the SPI was 1-5, where a higher score indicates more frequent performance. As can be surmised, program staff were least likely to perform services traditionally provided in the home of the elder including minor home repairs, budgeting assistance, laundry, cleaning, escort, friendly visiting, and bill paying/writing letters. On the other hand, services provided "often" to "very often" included meals, companionship, personal help with bathing, eating, dressing and toileting, simple nursing tasks, help with family problems, recreational activities, identifying client needs, speaking on behalf of the client at community offices, and providing emotional support.

Of course, day care activities may be provided by ADC program staff or by contracting with a provider. Table 2 presents data documenting the frequency with which a wide range of professional and supportive services were provided by staff as opposed to outsider contractees (these items were drawn from a composite measure of activity previously developed by the National Council on the Aging in their 1985 national survey (Von Behren, 1985). As shown, ADC programs in Pennsylvania more likely than not contract out for medically related services including M.D. assessment and treatment, psychiatry, podiatry, dentistry, physical, occupational and speech therapies, and transportation. On the other hand, their own staff carry the responsibility in most cases for the provision of social services, nursing, diet counseling, recreational activities, art and music therapy, exercises, reality therapy, meals, personal help with toileting, and field trips.

Other data not reported in Table 2 document several varieties of caregiver support services offered with varying frequency by ADC programs. Approximately 40% of the programs surveyed currently operate caregiver support groups. And, the majority of those who did not at the time of the survey indicated that they had plans to

TABLE 1. Frequency of Service Provision by ADC Programs

Service	Mean	S.D.
Meal Planning and/or Preparation	2.63	1.50
Serve-A-Meal	1.31	.75
Marketing or Shopping	3.78	.17
Household Cleaning	4.73	.90
Laundry	4.16	1.16
Escort	3.58	1.54
Companionship	2.04	1.49
Personal Help with Bathing, Eating, Dressing, Toileting	1.84	1.16
Simple Nursing Tasks	2.11	1.31
Budget Assistance	4.22	1.01
Teaching Proper Nutrition	2.59	1.04
Helping with Family Problems	1.93	.92
Recreational Activities	1.23	.68
Minor Home Repairs	4.95	.23
Friendly Visiting	3.55	1.36
Identifying Clients' Needs	1.17	.43
Speaking on Behalf of Clients at Community Offices	2.27	1.12
Providing Emotional Support	1.09	.34
Paying Bills/Writing Letters	3.91	1.03
SUMMARY INDEX SCORE	2.74	.54

Index Range: 1 - 5; where 1 = very often, 2 = often, 3 = sometimes, 4 = seldom, and 5 = never.

Summary Index Score Range: 1 - 5; where a higher score indicates less frequent performance.

TABLE 2. Adult Day Care Staff-Provided And Contracted Program Activities

Program Activity	Staff-Provided Activity		Contracted Activity	
	N	%	N	%
Social Services	39	70.9	16	29.1
M.D. Assessment	6	25.0	18	75.0
M.D. Treatment	4	25.0	12	75.0
Psychiatry	5	26.3	14	73.7
Podiatry	6	26.1	17	73.9
Dentistry	5	31.3	11	68.8
Nursing	35	85.4	6	14.6
Diet Counseling	27	77.1	8	22.9
Physical Therapy	9	27.3	24	72.7
Occupational Therapy	11	35.5	20	64.5
Speech Therapy	7	24.1	22	75.9
Recreational Activities	56	100.0	0	0.0
Art Therapy	34	73.9	12	26.1
Music Therapy	41	80.4	10	19.6
Exercises	58	100.0	0	0.0
Reality Therapy	53	96.4	2	3.6
Transportation (Home-Center)	7	14.0	43	86.0
Transportation-Other	10	25.0	30	75.0
Meals at Center	31	56.4	24	43.6
Toileting	57	100.0	0	0.0
Field Trips	48	72.7	0	18.2

organize such groups in the future. Fifty-four percent of the programs surveyed provided one-on-one counseling for family caregivers, while 30%-40% offered either informational meetings or annual program open houses for informal supports.

THE BENEFITS OF ADC

In the final analysis, the merits of ADC are perhaps best determined by data reflecting the degree and quality of personal satisfaction and program impact experienced by the formal and informal networks which provide services and receive services during daily program operations. Early, the potential for ADC to forestall institutionalization, provide less costly care for the infirm elderly, and possibly prolong life were documented (Ohnsorg, 1981; Wilson, 1984; Von Behren, 1989). What was the experience in Pennsylvania? Were clients satisfied with the service they received? Did ADC reduce caregiver stress? Were ADC directors and AAA program managers generally satisfied with the program? Was institutionalization delayed or avoided?

An Index of Consumer Satisfaction previously developed by Kaye (1982) was used to measure consumer views on the quality of service delivery. Both elder consumers and their informal caregivers were asked about their perceptions of staff sensitivity, respectfulness, and competency, as well as their overall satisfaction with the service. Their responses are presented in Table 3. Cronbach alphas (r) for client and informal caregiver responses on this index were .88 and .93 respectively, confirming high levels of internal consistency among index items. As shown, both clients and caregivers expressed high levels of satisfaction with ADC service. Interestingly, male elders emerged as experiencing significantly higher levels of program satisfaction than females (t = 3.67, p < .007).

In accordance with findings from other studies of ADC programming, the vast majority of informal caregivers felt they had experienced reduced stress (97% indicated this was the case) since their elder relatives had begun receiving ADC services. Stress reduction was usually experienced in the form of gains realized in personal

TABLE 3. Client and Caregiver Satisfaction With ADC Program (Satisfaction Index)

	Client		Caregiver	
	Mean	S.D.	Mean	S.D.
Were staff sensitive to client concerns?	4.39	.93	4.62	.68
Were staff respectful to client?	4.50	.67	4.71	.52
Were staff interested in the client?	4.54	.54	4.68	.53
Was client satisfied with services?	4.40	.96	4.68	.66
Were staff competent in dealing with client problems?	4.41	.75	4.59	.74
SUMMARY INDEX SCORE	4.48	.64	4.66	.56

Index score range was 1-5: where 1=strongly disagree; 2=disagree; 3=undecided; 4=agree; and 5=strongly agree.

Potential summary score range 1-5: where a higher score indicates a greater degree of satisfaction.

time, opportunities to return to the workplace, and relief from worry.

It is noteworthy, that both service recipients and their caregivers as well as staff in the Pennsylvania study emphasized difficulties pertaining to arranging for transportation services for elder consumers as being among the more problematic aspects of ADC. This particular feature of ADC programming appears to frequently emerge as challenging in operationalizing the ADC concept in many regions of the country.

SOCIAL WORK PRACTICE AND ADC

There is much evidence to suggest that ADC programming generally, and specifically those programs which are being funded through AAAs, are critically in need of the functional orientation and technical skills of the professional social worker. Indeed, Mace and Rabins (1984) found that social workers and nurses were the most commonly reported paid professional day care staff members and were most often the program directors of these projects. Furthermore, social services appear to be a central component of ADC initiatives, whether or not such programs claim to be influenced in their design by a medical or social model of care.

Social workers, as care managers, assess individual participant needs, coordinate care plans, and supervise services. These functions are essential to ADC programming. Social workers also assure appropriate counseling expertise based on their knowledge of aging, the emotional and social aspects of chronic illness, family dynamics, and the variety of additional community and institutional resources that are available. Indeed, the provision of personal care represents one of the core skill areas for the social work practitioner (Morris and Anderson, 1975). The social worker, in bringing this knowledge to ADC programs becomes a critical link in assuring quality of care (Huttman, 1985).

Findings from the Pennsylvania evaluation reported in this article confirmed that ADC primarily serves a respite and socialization function. Even so, when elder clients were asked what services they wished were more frequently available at the ADC program, the most frequently requested additional services were counseling-related. Such assistance was asked for by 31% of the elder clients who were interviewed. Furthermore, social services already represent one of the most common "staff-provided" as opposed to "contracted activity" according to ADC directors as reflected in the Pennsylvania study. Approximately seven in ten ADC programs had their own in-house staff provide social services. Identifying client needs, providing emotional support, and helping with family problems (three commonly identified social service-related functions) were among the most frequently delivered services by the Pennsylvania ADC programs which were surveyed. Needs identification and the provision of emotional support were, in fact, delivered more often than meals and recreational programming during the average day and represented the first and second most common tasks performed by staff (see Table 1). Even so, only half of these projects offered individual counseling services for family caregivers of the elderly attending ADC.

POLICY IMPLICATIONS AND RECOMMENDATIONS

Findings from the Pennsylvania evaluation of ADC combined with results from analyses of ADC performed elsewhere serve to confirm the desirability of this service intervention. The substantial growth over a relatively short period of time in this category of gerontological service perhaps best testifies to its popularity.

As ADC continues to evolve, program planners and policymakers in the gerontological services arena are likely to be increasingly pressed to establish formal policy and program standards which will assure consistent development and quality care by all ADC initiatives. Among their concerns should be advocating for the establishment and improvement of transportation services as well as the training of transportation staff in the needs of the frail elderly. Insuring the presence of adequate numbers of trained staff and specifically the availability of personnel able to provide professional counseling and caregiver support services for ADC clients and their families are essential as well.

Taken together, the formalization of these and other program standards will serve to maximize ADC's capacity to help frail older adults and their informal supports gain a measure of control over their personal environment and well-being while remaining outside the walls of institutional long-term care.

REFERENCES

Aaronson, L. (1983). Adult day care: A developing concept. *Journal of Gerontological Social Work*, 5, 3, 35-47.
Adult Day Care: A Community-Based Long-Term Care Option. (1983). Harrisburg, PA: Pennsylvania Council on Aging.
Arling, G. & Romaniuk, M. (1982). *Adult day care programs in Virginia.* Richmond, VA: Virginia Center on Aging, Virginia Commonwealth University.

Bilitski, J.S. (1985). Assessment of adult day care programs and client health characteristics in U.S. Region III. Diss. West Virginia University.

Bilitski, J.S. (1983). A process and product evaluation model of an adult day care center with implementation of process evaluation. Monesson, PA: Mon Valley Health and Welfare Council, Area Agency on Aging.

Bilitski, J.S. (1982). Nursing teaching, practice, and research in an adult day care center. Morgantown, WV: West Virginia University School of Nursing.

Carey, B. & Hanson, S. (1985/86). Social work groups with institutionalized Alzheimer's disease victims. *Journal of Gerontological Social Work*, 9, 2, 15-25.

Crossman, L. (1987). Adult day care: Coming of age. *The Aging Connection*, 8, 4, 1,3.

Harder, W.P., Gornick, J.C., & Burt, M.R. (1983). *Adult Day Care: Supplement or Substitute?* Draft Report. Washington, DC: The Urban Institute.

Hooyman, N. & Lustbader, W. (1986). *Taking Care.* New York: The Free Press.

Huttman, E. (1985). *Social Services for the Elderly.* New York: The Free Press.

Kane, R. & Kane, R. (1987). *Long-Term Care: Principles, Programs, and Policies.* New York: Springer Publishing Company.

Kaye, L.W. (1982). Home care services for older people: An organizational analysis of provider experience. Diss. Columbia University.

Kaye, L.W. & Kirwin, P.M. (1989). *An Evaluation of Adult Day Care Programs in Pennsylvania.* Final report prepared for the Pennsylvania Department of Aging. Bryn Mawr, PA: Bryn Mawr Graduate School of Social Work and Social Research.

Kirwin, P.M. (1989). An examination of the relationship between formal and informal systems in the service of adult day care for the frail elderly. Diss. Bryn Mawr College.

Kirwin, P.M. (1988). Correlates of service utilization among adult day care clients. *Home Health Care Services Quarterly*, 9, 1, 103-15.

Kirwin, P.M. (1986). Adult day care: An integrated model. In R. Dobrof (Ed.). *Social Work and Alzheimer's Disease.* New York: Haworth Press.

Koenen, R.E. (1980). Adult day care: A northwest perspective. *Journal of Gerontological Nursing*, 6, 4, 218-21.

Larmer, K. (1988). *Memorandum.* Washington, DC: National Council on the Aging, Inc.

Mace, N.L. & Rabins, P.V. (1984). *A Survey of Day Care for the Demented Adult in the United States.* Washington, DC: National Council on the Aging, Inc.

McCuan, E. & Elliott, M. (1977). Geriatric day care in theory and practice. *Social Work in Health Care*, 2, 153-70.

Mehta, N. & Mack, C. (1975). Day care services: An alternative to institutional care. *Journal of the American Geriatric Society*, 23, 6, 280-83.

Melcher, J. (1988). Toward expanded adult day care. *News Release.* Washington, DC: Senate Special Committee on Aging.

Morris, R. & Anderson, D. (1975). Personal care services: An identity for social work. *Social Service Review*, 49, 2, 157-74.

Ohnsorg, D.W. (1981). Burgeoning day care movement prolongs independent living. *Perspective on Aging*, X, 1, 18-20.

Padula, H. (1983). *Developing Adult Day Care: An Approach to Maintaining Independence for Impaired Older Persons*. Washington, DC: National Council on the Aging, Inc.

Rhodes, L.M. (1982). *A Weissert Profile and Functional Task Analysis of Vintage, Inc. Adult Day Care (Pittsburgh, PA)*. Washington, DC: Transcentury Corporation.

Smyer, M. (1980). The differential usage of services by impaired elderly. *Journal of Gerontology*, 35, 2, 249-255.

Stassen, M. & Holahan, J. (1981). *Long-Term Care Demonstration Projects: A Review of Recent Evaluations*. Washington, DC: The Urban Institute, 230.

Von Behren, R. (1989). Adult day care: A decade of growth. *Perspective on Aging*, XVIII, 4, 14-18.

Von Behren, R. (1988). *Adult Day Care: A Program of Services for the Functionally Impaired*. Washington, DC: National Institute on Adult Daycare, National Council on the Aging, Inc.

Weissert, W. (1975). *Adult day care in the United States: A comparative study: Final report*. Washington, DC: Transcentury.

Weissert, W. (1976). Two models of geriatric day care: Findings from a comparative study. *The Gerontologist*, 16, 5, 420-27.

Weissert, W. (1977). *Adult day care in the United States: Current research projects and a survey of 10 centers*. Public Health Reports, 92.

Weissert, W., Wan, T., and Livieratos, B. (1979). *Effects and costs of day care and homemaker services for the chronically ill: A randomized experiment. Executive summary*. Washington, DC: National Center for Health Services, U.S. Dept. of Health , Education, and Welfare.

Wilson, A.J. (1984). *Social Services for Older Persons*. Boston, MA: Little, Brown and Company.